UNIT 2

DIET AND NUTRITION ACTIVITIES

PATRICIA RIZZO TONER

Just for the HEALTH of It!
Health Curriculum Activities Library

THE CENTER FOR APPLIED
RESEARCH IN EDUCATION
West Nyack, New York 10995

Library of Congress Cataloging-in-Publication Data

Toner, Patricia Rizzo, 1952–
    Diet and nutrition activities / Patricia Rizzo Toner.
      p.   cm.—(Just for the health of it! : unit 2)
    "Includes 90 ready-to-use worksheets for grades 7–12."
    ISBN 0-87628-265-6
    1. Nutrition—Study and teaching (Secondary)   I. Title.
  II. Series.
  QP143.T65   1993   93-4965
  613.2′071′2—dc20   CIP

Printed in the United States of America

10   9   8

The source for many of the clip art images in this book is Presentation Task Force, a registered trademark of New Vision Technologies, Inc., copyright 1991.

ISBN 0-87628-265-6

**THE CENTER FOR APPLIED RESEARCH
IN EDUCATION**
West Nyack, NY 10994

On the World Wide Web at http://www.phdirect.com

DEDICATION

To my roommates at Trenton State College:

Kathy Asson Costello
Barb Cook Bruchac
Pat Minnick Stratton
Lorraine Koegler Harnish
Robin Sheppard

This dedication is in appreciation for the years of pure fun that we were able to share. As the years pass (a little more quickly than I'd like), I've come to realize just how special that time was.

As for dedicating a nutrition book. . .it's because nobody could cook a turkey like we could, and nobody could

forget to defrost it;
serve the vegetables at 5:00, and
serve the turkey itself at 9:00, while our dinner guest, the little old lady across the hall, adjusted her clock for four hours.

Thanks for the great times. May you and your families always find peace and happiness.

ACKNOWLEDGMENTS

Thanks, once again, to Barb Snyder and Colleen Leh of Holland Junior High, Holland, Pennsylvania, for reviewing each activity and providing valuable feedback.

Thanks to Marge Hunter of Holland Junior High, Holland, Pennsylvania, for her expertise in the areas of home economics, diet, and nutrition. Thanks, also, for valuable suggestions and review of the materials.

Thanks to school nurses Vivian Haines and Janet Ostoyich for suggestions and materials. A special thanks for help with the "Full of Baloney" activity.

Thanks to Shanna Mountford, Holland, Pennsylvania, for cutting and pasting the "Food Cards."

Thanks to Janet Borradaile, Holland, Pennsylvania, for cutting and pasting the "Food Playing Cards."

ABOUT THE AUTHOR

Patricia Rizzo Toner, M.Ed., has taught Health and Physical Education in the Council Rock School District, Holland, PA, for over 19 years, and she has also coached gymnastics and field hockey. She is the co-author of three books: *What Are We Doing in Gym Today?, You'll Never Guess What We Did in Gym Today!,* and *How to Survive Teaching Health.* Besides her work as a teacher, Pat is also a freelance cartoonist. A member of the American Alliance for Health, Physical Education, Recreation and Dance, Pat received the Hammond Service Award, the Marianna G. Packer Book Award and was named to *Who's Who Among Students in American Colleges and Universities,* as well as *Who's Who in American Education.*

ABOUT JUST FOR THE HEALTH OF IT!

Just for the Health of It! was developed to give you, the health teacher, new ways to present difficult-to-teach subjects and to spark your students' interest in day-to-day health classes. It includes over 540 ready-to-use activities organized for your teaching convenience into six separate, self-contained units focusing on six major areas of health education.

Each unit provides ninety classroom-tested activities printed in a full-page format and ready to be photocopied as many times as needed for student use. Many of the activities are illustrated with cartoon figures to enliven the material and help inject a touch of humor into the health curriculum.

The following briefly describes each of the six units in the series:

Unit 1: *Consumer Health and Safety Activities* helps students recognize advertising techniques, compare various products and claims, understand consumer rights, distinguish between safe and dangerous items, become familiar with safety rules, and more.

Unit 2: *Diet and Nutrition Activities* focuses on basic concepts and skills such as the four food groups, caloric balance or imbalance, the safety of diets, food additives, and vitamin deficiency diseases.

Unit 3: *Relationships and Communication Activities* explores topics such as family relationships, sibling rivalry, how to make friends, split-level communications, assertiveness and aggressiveness, dating, divorce, and popularity.

Unit 4: *Sex Education Activities* teaches about the male and female reproductive systems, various methods of contraception ranging from abstinence to mechanical and chemical methods, sexually transmitted diseases, the immune system, pregnancy, fetal development, childbirth, and more.

Unit 5: *Stress-Management and Self-Esteem Activities* examines the causes and signs of stress and teaches ways of coping with it. Along with these, the unit focuses on various elements of building self-esteem such as appearance, values, self-concept, success and confidence, personality, and character traits.

Unit 6: *Substance Abuse Prevention Activities* deals with the use and abuse of tobacco, alcohol, and other drugs and examines habits ranging from occasional use to addiction. It also promotes alternatives to drug use by examining peer pressure situations, decision-making, and where to seek help.

To help you mix and match activities from the series with ease, all of the activities in each unit are designated with two letters to represent each resource as follows: Sex Education (SE), Substance Abuse Prevention (SA), Relationships and Communication (RC), Stress-Management and Self-Esteem (SM), Diet and Nutrition (DN), and Consumer Health and Safety (CH).

About Unit 2

Diet and Nutrition Activities provides you with many activities for your Nutrition unit.

This resource is designed for busy teachers who are looking to enhance their collection of materials, activities, and ideas. It contains two main teaching tools:

- reproducibles designed for quick copying to hand out to students; and
- activities that give you ideas, games, and instructions to enhance your classroom presentation.

Use these ideas to introduce a Diet and Nutrition unit, to increase interest at any given point in a lesson, or to reinforce knowledge.

An at-a-glance table of contents provides valuable help by supplying general and specific topic heads with a complete listing of activities and reproducibles. The ninety activities that make up this resource focus on the following important elements of diet and nutrition.

Systems of the Body. This section covers the digestive system and its accessory organs and glands, as well as the muscular system.

Essential Nutrients. The many games and activities in this section deal with the body's need for protein, fats, carbohydrates, vitamins, minerals, and water.

Meeting Nutritional Needs. Learn about the food groups by playing a variety of games such as CONCENTRATION and GO FISH! This section includes the Food Playing Cards that can be used in numerous ways.

Consumer Awareness. Understand the new Food Guide Pyramid, the U.S. RDA, nutrition labeling, unit pricing, and open dating.

Food Safety. This section focuses on the use of and reasons for food additives, current consumer concerns, and food safety rules.

Eating Healthy. Learn about balancing your diet and limiting your intake of fats, sodium, cholesterol, and sugars. Find out about your snacking habits.

Factors Affecting Diet. This section deals with how factors like personal taste, family customs, emotions, and advertising affect our eating habits.

Weight Control. Activities and reproducibles in this section focus on caloric intake and expenditure, hazards of obesity, weight control hints, and dieting.

Eating Disorders. Understand what anorexia nervosa and bulimia can do to the body and research places to get help. Discuss the media's role in contributing to an unrealistic image of physical perfection.

The reproducibles and activities are designated *DN*, representing the Diet and Nutrition component of the *Health Curriculum Activities Library*. These games, activities, puzzles, charts, and worksheets can be put directly into your lesson plans. Use them on an individual basis or as a whole-class activity.

I hope you enjoy the materials in *Diet and Nutrition Activities*. Good luck!

Patricia Rizzo Toner

CONTENTS

SYSTEMS OF THE BODY

- **Digestive System**

- **Accessory Organs and Glands**

- **Muscular System**

BREAKDOWN (DN-1)

DIRECTIONS: The purpose of the digestive system is to break down food into simple molecules that pass into the bloodstream to provide the body with energy for life. Label the parts of the digestive system on the diagram below. Use the words in the box to help you.

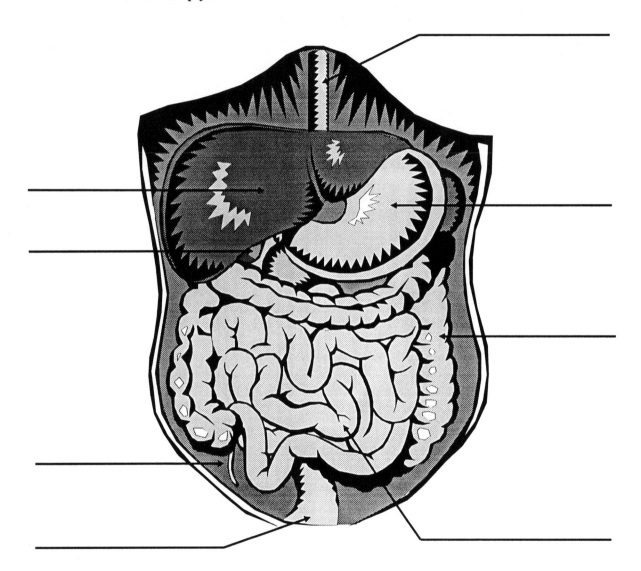

appendix	**large intestine**
gallbladder	**rectum**
liver	**esophagus**
stomach	**small intestine**

AS THE STOMACH CHURNS (DN-2)

DIRECTIONS: Label the parts of the digestive system shown below. Use the words in the box.

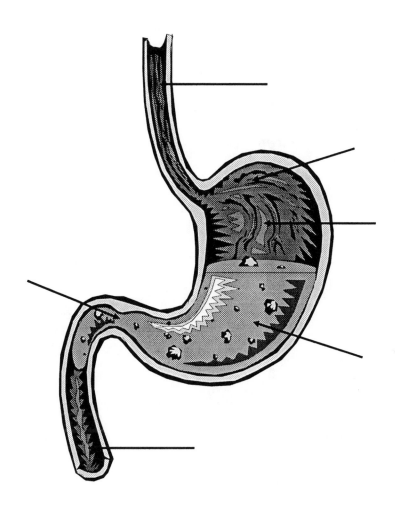

| esophagus |
| fundus |
| duodenum |
| pylorus |
| stomach |
| antrum |

Name _____   Date _____

LIVER, GALLBLADDER, AND PANCREAS (DN-3)

DIRECTIONS: The liver, gallbladder, and pancreas are aids in the digestive process. Read about their functions in the boxes, then label the parts using the words in the box at the bottom of the sheet.

Gallbladder:
The gallbladder is a small sac that stores bile. The gallbladder is located on the underside of the liver.

Pancreas:
The pancreas produces alkaline enzymes that flow into the small intestine. The pancreas also produces insulin and glucagon.

Liver:
The liver, the largest gland in the body, has over 500 functions. Its major functions are:
1. Production of bile, a yellowish-green fluid that helps to break down fats.
2. Conversion of glucose to glycogen.
3. Balance of blood sugar in the body.
4. Helping to metabolize carbohydrates, fats, and proteins.
5. Changing toxic wastes into less toxic substances.
6. Stores fat-soluble vitamins A, D, E, and K and several water-soluble vitamins.

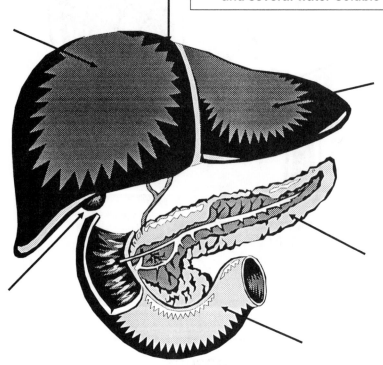

liver	left lobe
gallbladder	right lobe
pancreas	duodenum

Name _____   **Date** _____

MUSCLE HUSTLE (DN-4)

DIRECTIONS: Label the parts of the muscular system below, by using the words in the box.

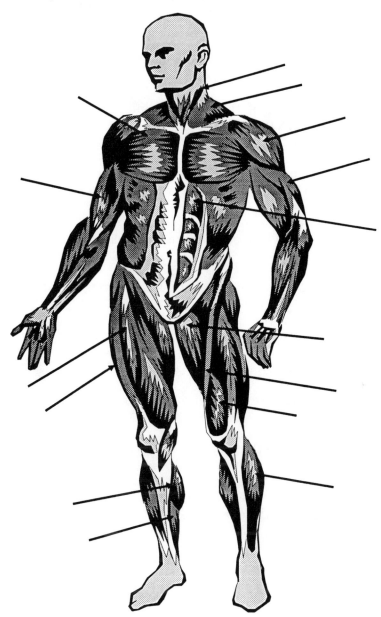

pectoralis major	**sternocleidomastoid**	**rectus femoris**
peroneus longus	**trapezius**	**vastus lateralis**
vastus medialis	**deltoid**	**gastrocnemius**
sartorius	**biceps**	**rectus abdominus**
soleus	**triceps**	**adductor longus**

MUSCLE MADNESS (DN-5)

DIRECTIONS: Unscramble the underlined words to complete these sentences about the muscular system. Write your answer in the blank to the left of each sentence.

_____ 1. Muscles that we can consciously move are called <u>RNOVLTUAY</u> muscles.

_____ 2. Shortening of the muscle that causes movement is called muscular <u>RACCONTTNIO</u>.

_____ 3. The muscles found in the walls of the stomach and intestines are called <u>MOOTHS</u> muscles.

_____ 4. <u>LEKSELTA</u> muscles are responsible for movement of the body and limbs.

_____ 5. The muscle that straightens the arm is called the <u>SCITREP</u>.

_____ 6. If the blood supply doesn't keep up with muscle activity, <u>UGTAFIE</u> is the result.

_____ 7. Muscles are connected to bones by <u>NENTOSD</u>.

_____ 8. The muscle that bends the arm at the elbow is the <u>SPCIBE</u>.

_____ 9. Skeletal muscles are attached to bones at two ends. One end is called the origin and the opposite end is the <u>NIESINTRO</u>.

_____ 10. The ability of a muscle to stay tense is known as muscle <u>NOTE</u>.

ESSENTIAL NUTRIENTS

- General

- Carbohydrates

- Fats

- Vitamins and Minerals

ACTIVITY 1: CATEGORIES

Concept/ Description: There are six essential nutrients that the body requires.

Objective: To be the first group to place all the foods in the proper nutrient categories.

Materials: Categories Game Cards (DN-7 to DN-11)
Categories Game Answer Key (DN-6)
Chalkboard
Chalk
Masking tape

Directions: 1. Photocopy two sets of the Categories Game Cards and cut the cards apart, being careful not to mix up the sets. (You may want to laminate the cards first for durability).

2. Shuffle each set of cards separately.

3. Write the following categories on the board as shown in Figure 1:

> Vitamins
>
> Minerals
>
> Proteins
>
> Carbohydrates
>
> Fats
>
> Water

4. Divide the class into two teams and assign each person on the team a number. Give each person a card, face down.

5. Have each person roll up a piece of masking tape and place it on the back of the card, so it will stick to the chalkboard.

6. On the signal, each team will send a team member to the board, one at a time, in numerical order, to stick his or her card on the board under the proper category heading. The next person may not go until the first is seated. If the card is placed in the incorrect category, the team may not correct it until all cards have been placed. At that time, one player, who has been designated team captain, may return to the board to change any cards. The captain may receive help from the team.

7. The first team to have all its members sitting in their assigned seats and all their cards in the correct categories is declared the winner.

CATEGORIES Game Answer Key (DN-6)

Vitamins
GRAPEFRUIT
BROCCOLI
SPINACH
TOMATO
LETTUCE
PINEAPPLE
CARROTS
CABBAGE
LEMON
MILK*
TURKEY
PORK CHOPS

Minerals
TABLE SALT
SHELLFISH
MILK*

Proteins
STEAK
EGG
ROAST BEEF
MAYONNAISE
SALAD DRESSING

Carbohydrates
CEREAL
BREAD
MACARONI
ROLL

Fats
MARGARINE
BUTTER
OIL

Water
TAP WATER
CRUSHED ICE
ICE CUBES
NATURAL SPRING WATER

MILK can go in either category, since it is a rich supply of both calcium and vitamin D.

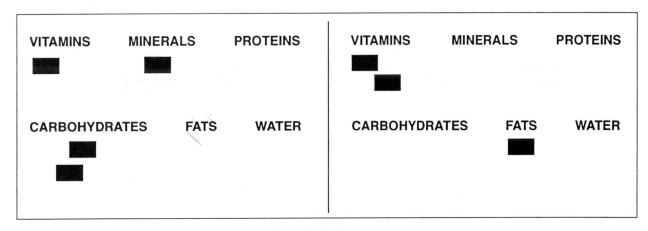

Figure 1. Blackboard set-up for CATEGORIES Game.

CATEGORIES Game Cards (DN-7)

GRAPEFRUIT	**BROCCOLI**
SPINACH	**TOMATO**
LETTUCE	**PINEAPPLE**

CARROTS	**CABBAGE**
LEMON	**TABLE SALT**
SHELLFISH	**MILK**

CATEGORIES Game Cards (DN-9)

STEAK	**EGG**
ROAST BEEF	**TURKEY**
PORK CHOPS	**CEREAL**

CATEGORIES Game Cards (DN-10)

BREAD	**MACARONI**
ROLL	**MARGARINE**
BUTTER	**OIL**

MAYONNAISE	**SALAD DRESSING**
TAP WATER	**CRUSHED ICE**
ICE CUBES	**NATURAL SPRING WATER**

Name _____   **Date** _____

CARBO CHARGED (DN-12)

Carbohydrates are starches and sugars that come mainly from plant food. Carbohydrates provide the body with much of the energy it needs each day. There are two types of carbohydrates: COMPLEX, or starches, and SIMPLE, or sugars.

DIRECTIONS: Fill in the words below to give some examples of some complex and simple carbohydrates.

Complex Carbohydrates:

1. _ _ S _ _ _ _
2. _ _ T _
3. _ A _ _ _ _
4. _ R _ _ _ _
5. C _ _ _ _ _
6. _ _ _ _ H _ _ _ _
7. _ _ E _ _
8. _ _ _ _ S

CLUES

1. Type of cooked potato
2. Type of pasta
3. Type of cooked potato
4. White, wheat, rye, etc.
5. Found on pizza, bread, rolls, etc.
6. Type of pasta
7. Type of whole-grain bread
8. Hard, dinner, crescent, etc.

CLUES

1. 7-Up, Coca-Cola, Mountain Dew, etc.
2. Refined, sweet substance found in the home
3. Kind of jelly
4. Kind of syrup
5. Fruit sugar
6. Milk sugar

Simple Carbohydrates:

1. S _ _ _   _ _ _ _ _ _
2. _ _ _ _ _ _U _ _ _
3. G _ _ _ _ _
4. _ A _ _ _ _
5. _ R _ _ _ _ _ _
6. _ _ _ _ _S _

Name _____ **Date** _____

FATTY BOOM-BA-LATTY (DN-13)

DIRECTIONS: For each item below, place an *X* in the box indicating which food you think contains more fat.

☐ 2 slices cheese pizza

☐ 1 fish sandwich

☐ 1 peanut butter and jelly sandwich

☐ 1 roasted pork chop

☐ 1 cup spaghetti and meatballs

☐ 1 small taco

☐ 10 french fries

☐ 10 baked potatoes

☐ 3 oz. fish sticks

☐ 2 sausage links

☐ 1/2 croissant

☐ 2 English muffins

☐ 1 regular cheeseburger

☐ 3 oz. sirloin steak

☐ 1/2 cup canned pudding

☐ 10-oz. vanilla milkshake

☐ 6 pancakes

☐ 1 cinnamon sweet roll

☐ 1 cup macaroni and cheese

☐ 10 slices bread

☐ 2 cups lowfat yogurt

☐ 1 tablespoon mayonnaise

☐ 1 oz. tortilla chips

☐ 1 cup unbuttered popcorn

FAT FACTS (DN-14)

DIRECTIONS: Find the letter that matches the number and fill it in on the blank line. Read the information about fat in the diet and discuss.

A	B	C	D	E	F	G	H	I	J	K	L	M
1	2	3	4	5	6	7	8	9	10	11	12	13

N	O	P	Q	R	S	T	U	V	W	X	Y	Z
14	15	16	17	18	19	20	21	22	23	24	25	26

The building blocks of fats are __ __ __ __ __ acids. There are three types:
6 1 20 20 25

monounsaturated, polyunsaturated, and __ __ __ __ __ __ __ __ __ . Fats that remain
19 1 20 21 18 1 20 5 4

__ __ __ __ __ __ at room temperature are either monounsaturated or polyunsaturated.
12 9 17 21 9 4

Some examples of polyunsaturated fats include oils made from __ __ __ __ safflower,
3 15 18 14

sunflower, __ __ __ __ __ __ __ cottonseed, and __ __ __ __ __ __ . Monounsaturated
19 15 25 2 5 1 14   19 5 19 1 13 5

oils are __ __ __ __ __ , canola, avocado, and __ __ __ __ __ __ .
15 12 9 22 5   16 5 1 14 21 20

More harmful because they cause the __ __ __ __ __ to produce too much
12 9 22 5 18

__ __ __ __ __ __ __ __ __ __ __ are saturated fats, which remain __ __ __ __ __
3 8 15 12 5 19 20 5 18 15 12   19 15 12 9 4

or semisolid at room temperature. Shortening and margarine are examples and are also referred

to as hydrogenated or partially hydrogenated. Many __ __ __ __ __ __ products are high in
1 14 9 13 1 12

saturated fats, such as __ __ __ __ , pork, lamb, butter, __ __ __ __ __ milk, and dairy
2 5 5 6   23 8 15 12 5

products from whole milk. Palm, palm-kernel, and __ __ __ __ __ __ __ oil are also high
3 15 3 15 14 21 20

in saturated fats.

It's best to __ __ __ down on __ __ __ the fats and oils we eat to lower our risk of
3 21 20   1 12 12

__ __ __ __ __ disease.
8 5 1 18 20

FOR YOUR INFORMATION (DN-15)

Listed below are some common foods, their calorie content, and the amount of fat in each. Compare the various foods. Are you surprised to find large amounts of fat in any of the foods?

FOOD	AMOUNT	CALORIES	FAT (g)
American Cheese	1 oz.	106	9
Cheddar Cheese	1 oz.	114	9
Cottage Cheese	1/2 cup	102	2
Mozzarella Cheese	1 oz.	72	5
Swiss Cheese	1 oz.	107	8
Ice Cream	1/2 cup	135	7
Ice Milk	1/2 cup	92	3
2% Chocolate Milk	1 cup	179	5
Skim Milk	1 cup	86	0
2% Lowfat Milk	1 cup	121	5
Whole Milk	1 cup	150	8
Chocolate Milkshake	10 oz.	360	11
Chocolate Pudding	1/2 cup	155	4
Frozen Yogurt	1/2 cup	225	3
Plain Yogurt	1 cup	144	4
Fried Chicken	3 oz.	218	11
Roasted Chicken	3 oz.	139	3
Ground Beef (broiled)	3 oz.	246	18
Baked Halibut	3 oz.	119	2
Baked Ham	3 oz.	156	9
Beef Hot Dog	2 oz.	184	17
Peanut Butter	2 tablespoons	188	16
Broiled Pork Chop	3 oz.	219	13
Roast Beef	3 oz.	164	7
Baked Potato	1 large	220	0
French Fries	10 strips	158	8
Bagel	1/2	100	1
Biscuit	1 small	95	3
Bran Muffin	1 small	140	4
Corn Flakes	1 oz.	110	0
Croissant	1/2 roll	118	6
English Muffin	1/2 muffin	70	1
Oatmeal (instant)	1/2 cup	73	1
Pancake	1	60	2
White Rice (cooked)	1/2 cup	131	0
White Bread	1 slice	65	1
Whole Wheat Bread	1 slice	70	1

FOR YOUR INFORMATION, TOO (DN-16)

Listed below are more common foods, their calorie content, and the amount of fat in each. Compare the various foods. Are you surprised to find large amounts of fat in any of these foods?

FOOD	AMOUNT	CALORIES	FAT (g)
Cheeseburger	1 regular	359	20
Cheese Pizza	2 slices	218	5
Fish Sandwich (with Cheese)	1 sandwich	524	29
Macaroni and Cheese	1 cup	430	22
Quiche (with bacon)	1/8 8-inch pie	342	26
Spaghetti and Meatballs	1 cup	330	12
Taco (with meat)	1 small	370	21
Apple Pie	1/8 9-inch pie	303	13
Corn Chips	1 oz.	155	9
Doughnut	1	210	12
Pretzels	1 oz.	112	1
Butter	1 tablespoon	102	12
Mayonnaise	1 tablespoon	99	11

ACTIVITY 2: FOOD DISPLAY

Concept/ Description: Vitamins and minerals play important roles in maintaining a healthy body.

Objective: To research various vitamins and minerals and their food sources and display the findings visually.

Materials: Will depend on type of project chosen.

Directions:
1. Assign each student, or group of students, a vitamin or mineral to research.
2. Ask students to determine the importance of that substance to maintaining good health. Also, list the foods that provide these nutrients.
3. Next, have students determine a way to display the results. Suggestions include mobiles, posters, charts, collages, or edible food models.
4. Display the finished projects around the room.

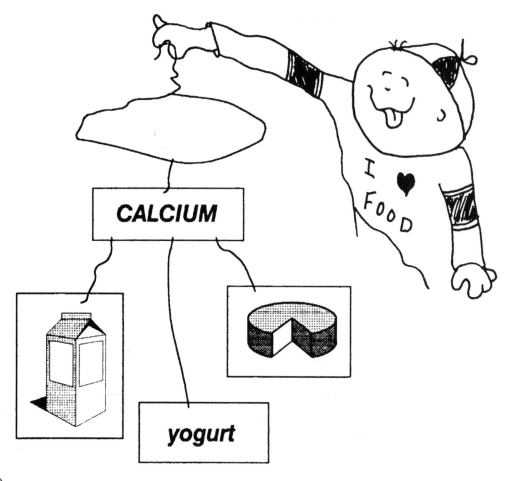

CALCIUM

yogurt

Name _____ **Date** _____

VITAMIN MATCH-UP (DN-17)

DIRECTIONS: Match the vitamin with its function by placing the name of the vitamin in the blank to the left. The vitamins are listed in the box.

B₁ (thiamine)	B₂ (riboflavin)	B₃ (niacin)	B₆ (pyridoxine)
B₁₂ (cobalamin)	folic acid	Biotin	pantothenic acid
C (ascorbic acid)	A	D	E K

_____ 1. Maintains healthy skin, bones, and eyes.

_____ 2. Aids in blood clotting.

_____ 3. Aids in the functioning of the digestive tract.

_____ 4. Aids in red blood cell formation and synthesis of RNA and DNA.

_____ 5. Aids in digestion and carbohydrate use and is necessary for functioning of the nervous system.

_____ 6. Aids in metabolizing carbohydrates and other B vitamins.

_____ 7. Aids in connective tissue, bone, tooth, and skin formation; resistance to infection; and iron assimilation.

_____ 8. Aids in protein, fat, and carbohydrate metabolism.

_____ 9. Aids in energy production in cells; promotes healthy skin.

_____10. Aids in blood cell formation, protein production, and enzyme functioning.

_____11. Aids in carbohydrate use; necessary for heart, nervous system, and appetite.

_____12. Aids in calcium and phosphorous use.

_____13. Aids in maintenance of vitamin A and fats.

PLUS AND MINUS (DN-18)

DIRECTIONS: Research the vitamins listed and write the problems that occur when there is a deficiency and an excess of each. Write your answers in the boxes. Note: In some cases, an excess of the vitamin does not cause problems, nor does it have any benefits. The body will rid itself of the excess.

VITAMIN	DEFICIENCY (−)	EXCESS (+)
A		
D		
K		UNKNOWN
Folic Acid		— — —
B6		— — —
B12		— — —
C		
Niacin		
Riboflavin		— — —
Thiamine		— — —

Name _____   **Date** _____

DISSOLVE IN WATER (DN-19)

There are two classes of vitamins: fat-soluble and water-soluble. Fat-soluble vitamins are stored by the body and can be harmful if consumed in excess. Water-soluble vitamins are not stored by the body, so it is important that you eat foods that supply these vitamins every day.

DIRECTIONS: Write the fat-soluble vitamins in the fat molecule and the water-soluble vitamins in the water drop. Then, list some foods that supply you with each vitamin.

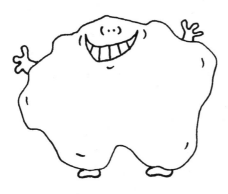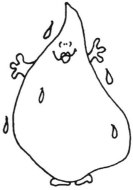

Vitamin A _____

Vitamin B_1 _____

Vitamin K _____

Vitamin B_{12} _____

Vitamin B_6 _____

Biotin _____

Vitamin C _____

Vitamin D _____

Vitamin E _____

Pantothenic Acid _____

Folic Acid _____

Vitamin B_2 _____

Vitamin B_3 _____

23

ACTIVITY 3: MATCHING MINERALS

**Concept/
Description:**   Minerals are essential to good health.

Objective: To be the first group to correctly match each mineral with its functions and food sources.

Materials: Matching Minerals Cards (DN-20)
Scissors

Directions: 1. Divide the class into groups of four.
2. Prior to class, photocopy one set of Matching Minerals cards for each group.
3. On the signal, each group tries to match the mineral (white cards) with its functions (medium gray cards) and its food sources (dark gray cards).
4. The first group to correctly match all minerals is the winner. NOTE: The minerals, their functions, and food sources are aligned properly on the following page. Keep an uncut copy for reference.

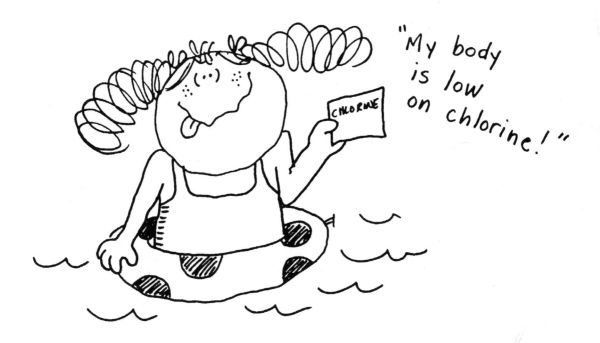

"My body is low on chlorine!"

MATCHING MINERALS Cards (DN-20)

CALCIUM	Aids in bone and tooth formation and blood clotting; needed for muscle and nerve activity	DAIRY PRODUCTS, DARK GREEN VEGETABLES, SARDINES
CHLORINE	Aids in digestion and water balance in the cells	TABLE SALT, MILK, MEAT, EGGS
MAGNESIUM	Maintains muscles and nerves; aids in metabolism	LEGUMES, NUTS, CHOCOLATE, WHOLE GRAINS, DARK GREEN VEGETABLES
PHOSPHOROUS	Aids bone and tooth formation and in maintenance of acid balance in blood	MEAT, EGGS, NUTS, FISH, POULTRY, WHOLE GRAINS
POTASSIUM	Helps to maintain heartbeat, water balance, and nerve transmission; aids in metabolism	ORANGE JUICE, CITRUS FRUITS, BANANAS, GREEN LEAFY VEGETABLES
SODIUM	Helps to maintain water balance; aids in nerve and muscle transmissions	TABLE SALT, SHELLFISH, ORGAN MEATS, CARROTS, BEETS
IRON	Prevents anemia; forms a part of hemoglobin	LIVER, RED MEAT, EGGS, GREEN LEAFY VEGETABLES
IODINE	Essential for normal metabolism; part of thyroid hormone	SEAFOOD, ADDED TO SALT

CONSUMER AWARENESS

- **Food Groups**

- **Food Guide Pyramid**

- **U.S. Recommended Daily Allowances**

- **Nutrition Labeling**

- **Shopping**

Name _____   **Date** _____

JOIN THE GROUP (DN-21)

DIRECTIONS: Color the foods below according to their food group. Follow the color code given.

COLOR CODE:

Fats, Oils, Sweets	Yellow
Milk, Yogurt, Cheese	Tan
Vegetables	Green
Fruits	Red
Grains	Brown
Meat, Poultry, Fish, Dry Beans, Eggs, Nuts	Blue

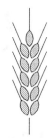

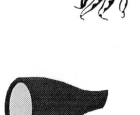
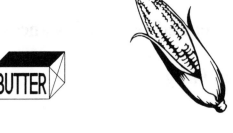
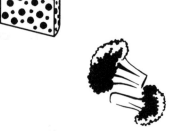
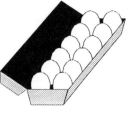

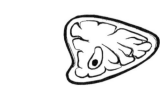
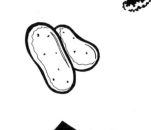
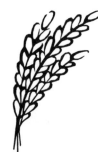
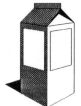
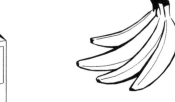

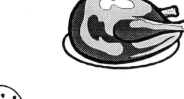

Name _____ **Date** _____

ONE-DAY FOOD DIARY (DN-22)

DIRECTIONS: Write down all the foods you eat for one day. Fill in the chart by writing an *X* in the appropriate food group column. Did you eat at least the minimum recommended servings for each food group?

FOOD OR DRINK	AMOUNT	DAIRY	MEAT	FRUIT	VEGE-TABLE	GRAIN	FATS,OILS, SWEETS
Total servings for the day							
Recommended minimum number of servings		2	2	2	3	6	███
Additional servings needed							

ANATOMY OF A LUNCH (DN-23)

DIRECTIONS: Look at the lunch below. Next to each item, place the name of the food group to which each food belongs.

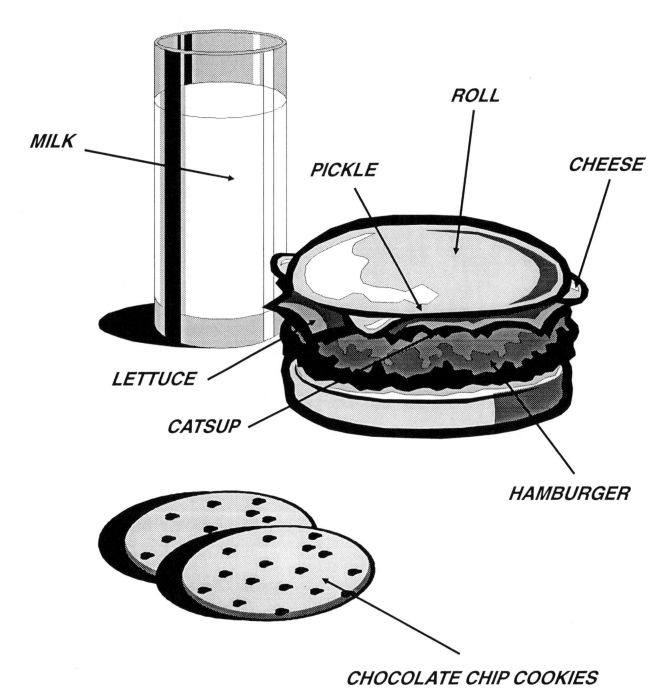

ROLL

MILK

PICKLE

CHEESE

LETTUCE

CATSUP

HAMBURGER

CHOCOLATE CHIP COOKIES

ACTIVITY 4: RECIPE RAIDERS

**Concept/
Description:** Some recipes contain foods from all the food groups and some are lacking in certain groups.

Objective: To analyze recipes and see what can be added to make a meal that has foods from all food groups.

Materials: Recipe Analysis Chart (DN-24)
Recipes
Pen or pencil

Directions:
1. Have students ask their parents for a copy of a favorite dinner recipe and bring it to class.
2. Using the Recipe Analysis Chart, have students determine which food groups are represented and which are not.
3. Ask students to add foods to a menu to provide a balanced meal.

Variations:
1. You provide the recipes and reproduce enough copies for each class member. Discuss as a class.
2. Speak to the Home Economics teacher. Perhaps a Home Ec class can make a balanced recipe for all to sample.
3. Put the recipes together into a recipe booklet, decorate it, include some nutrition information that you have studied in class, and have students give the completed book to their parents.

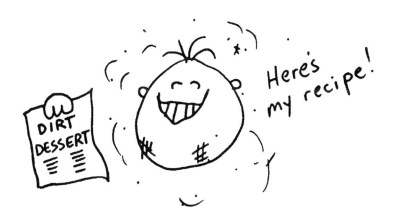

Name _____   **Date** _____

RECIPE ANALYSIS CHART (DN-24)

DIRECTIONS: Check your recipe to see if it has foods from all the food groups. Write each ingredient in the proper space. Answer the questions at the bottom.

GROUP	*INGREDIENTS*
Meat Group	
Fruits	
Vegetables	
Grain Group	
Milk Group	
Fats, Oils, Sweets	

©1993 by The Center for Applied Research in Education

1. Does your recipe have foods from all food groups?

2. What could you serve with this meal to have foods from all groups?

ACTIVITY 5: FAVORITE FOODS

**Concept/
Description:** It is important to eat a variety of foods from all the food groups to maintain a balanced diet.

Objective: For students to determine if they eat foods from all the food groups.

Materials: Favorite Foods Fold-Out (DN-25)
Scissors
Pen or pencil

Directions:
1. Photocopy the Favorite Foods Fold-Out and give one to each student.
2. Have students circle all the foods they like.
3. When they are finished, have the students cut out the box containing the food names.
4. Have students fold the paper lengthwise and crease it. Then fold the paper into thirds and crease it.
5. When the paper is unfolded, it should form six boxes representing the food groups.
6. Ask students which food groups have the most items circled.
7. Discuss ways to balance a diet that is unbalanced. Discuss the importance of a balanced diet.

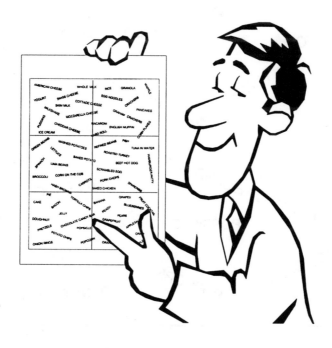

FAVORITE FOODS FOLD-OUT (DN-25)

AMERICAN CHEESE

WHOLE MILK

RICE

GRANOLA

WAFFLE

YOGURT

SWISS CHEESE

EGG NOODLES

CRACKERS

COTTAGE CHEESE

SKIM MILK

PANCAKES

MILKSHAKE

MOZZARELLA CHEESE

GRAHAM CRACKERS

PUDDING

CORN FLAKES

MACARONI

ENGLISH MUFFIN

CHEDDAR CHEESE

ICE CREAM

HARD ROLL

GREEN BEANS

MASHED POTATOES

REFRIED BEANS

FISH

TUNA IN WATER

LETTUCE

ROASTED TURKEY

BAKED POTATO

BEEF HOT DOG

SPINACH

LIMA BEANS

SCRAMBLED EGG

HAMBURGER PATTY

BROCCOLI

CORN ON THE COB

PORK CHOPS

CARROTS

SPARERIBS

HASH BROWNS

BAKED CHICKEN

PIE

GRAPES

FRUIT COCKTAIL

CAKE

TORTILLA CHIPS

BANANA

BLUEBERRIES

BACON

PEACH

JELLY

PEARS

DOUGHNUT

CHOCOLATE CANDY BAR

GRAPEFRUIT

APPLESAUCE

PRETZELS

POPSICLE

STRAWBERRIES

ORANGES

POTATO CHIPS

ONION RINGS

POPCORN

ORANGE JUICE

APPLE

ACTIVITY 6: CONCENTRATION

Concept/Description: Students will play the popular game, Concentration, by matching cards from the same food group.

Objective: To be the player to match the most cards.

Materials: Food Playing Cards (DN-26 to DN-31)
3-inch by-5-five-inch index cards (optional)
Paste or glue (optional)
Scissors
Large playing surface (desk, table, floor)

Directions:
1. Reproduce one set of Food Playing Cards per group of four players. Cut the cards apart and mount on index cards with paste or glue, or laminate the cards so they can be used repeatedly. Pick six cards from each food group and place them face down in a six-by-six grid in front of the group.

2. The first player turns over any two cards. If both foods are from the same food group, that player takes the two cards as a "match." If not, the cards are turned back over and the next player goes.

3. Play continues until all cards are matched. The person with the most cards is the winner.

Variations:
1. Play in teams, with teammates permitted to confer on which cards to turn over. The play proceeds from team to team and the team with the most cards is the winner.

2. Enlarge the cards and tape them to the wall or chalkboard so the whole class can see. Tape a piece of paper over each card and number the papers from 1 to 36. Divide the class into two teams. Team A calls out two numbers which are turned over (the paper is flipped up). If both foods are from the same food group, the team gets the cards. If not, the card is covered again. Team B then proceeds. Play continues until all the cards are matched, and the team with more is the winner.

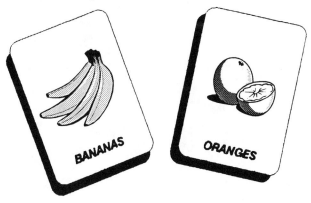

ACTIVITY 7: GO FISH!

Concept/
Description: Students will play the popular card game, Go Fish, by matching cards from the same food group.

Objective: To be the first player to match all cards and have no playing cards in his or her hands.

Materials: Food Playing Cards (DN-26 to DN-31)
3-inch by 5-inch index cards (optional)
Paste or glue (optional)
Scissors

Directions:
1. Reproduce one set of Food Playing Cards per group of three players. Cut the cards apart and mount on index cards with paste or glue, or laminate the cards so they can be used repeatedly.

2. Divide the class into groups of three and give each group a set of cards.

3. Deal seven cards, face down, to each player and put the remaining cards face down to form a draw pile.

4. If players have two foods from the same food group, they place them down as a match.

5. In turn, each player asks the player to the left for all the foods from a certain food group. For example, Tom might say to Jamie, "Give me all your Grains." If Jamie has cards from the Grain Group, she must give all of them to Tom. If not, Jamie says, "Go Fish." Tom then has to draw from the draw pile.

6. Play continues until a player has matched all of the cards and has none left in his/her hand. That person is declared the winner.

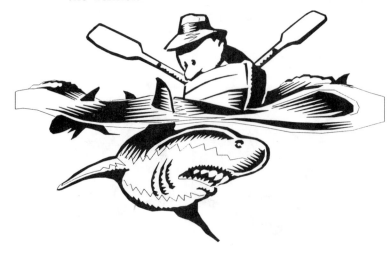

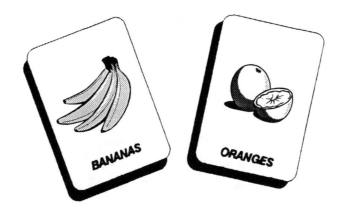

FOOD PLAYING CARDS

The following food playing cards are for use with Go Fish! and Concentration, and can be used in many other creative ways. Have students make up their own card games or adapt other card games.

The cards are placed in their respective food groups for your convenience.

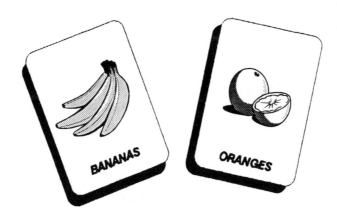

MILK, YOGURT, AND CHEESE Playing Cards (DN-26)

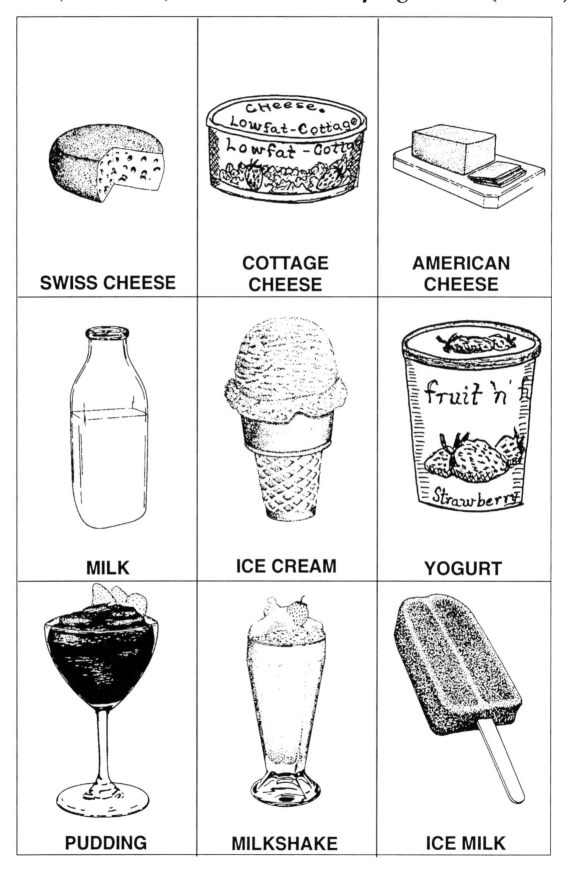

SWISS CHEESE	**COTTAGE CHEESE**	**AMERICAN CHEESE**
MILK	**ICE CREAM**	**YOGURT**
PUDDING	**MILKSHAKE**	**ICE MILK**

FRUIT Playing Cards (DN-27)

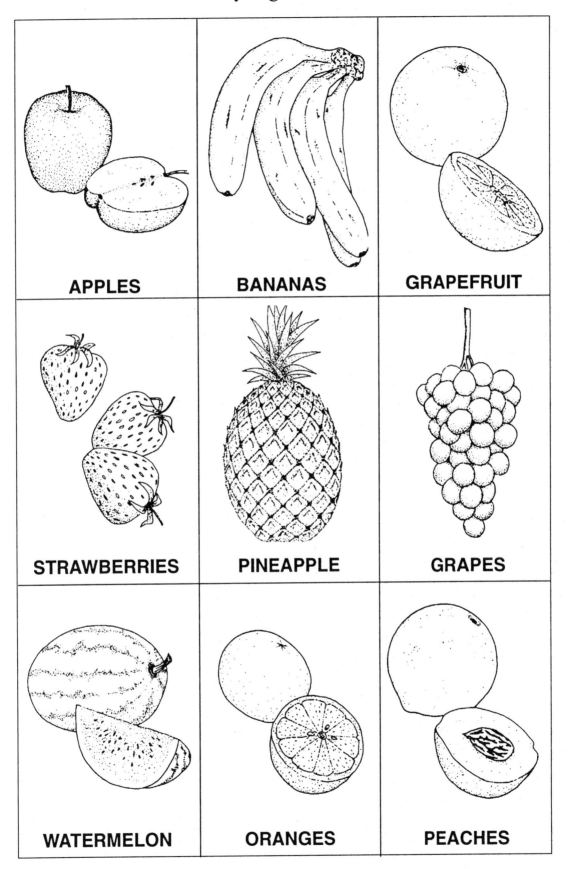

APPLES	**BANANAS**	**GRAPEFRUIT**
STRAWBERRIES	**PINEAPPLE**	**GRAPES**
WATERMELON	**ORANGES**	**PEACHES**

FATS, OILS, AND SWEETS Playing Cards (DN-28)

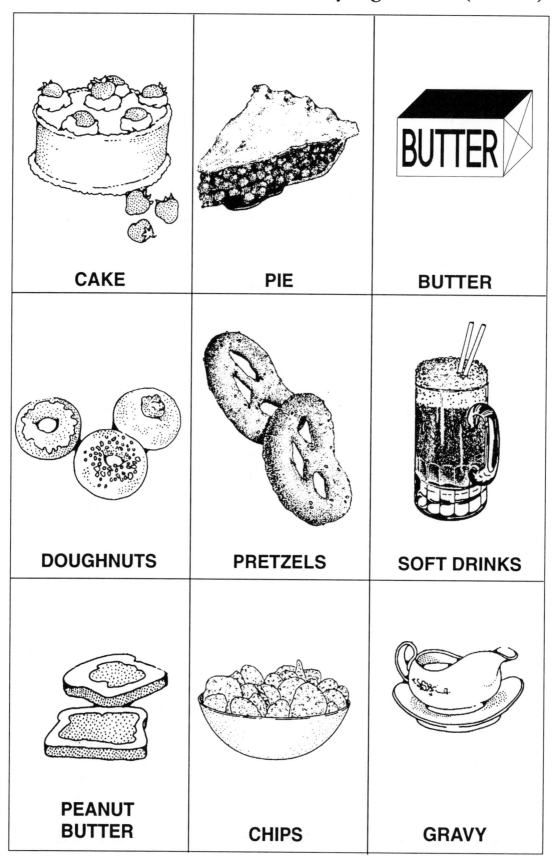

CAKE	PIE	BUTTER
DOUGHNUTS	PRETZELS	SOFT DRINKS
PEANUT BUTTER	CHIPS	GRAVY

VEGETABLE Playing Cards (DN-29)

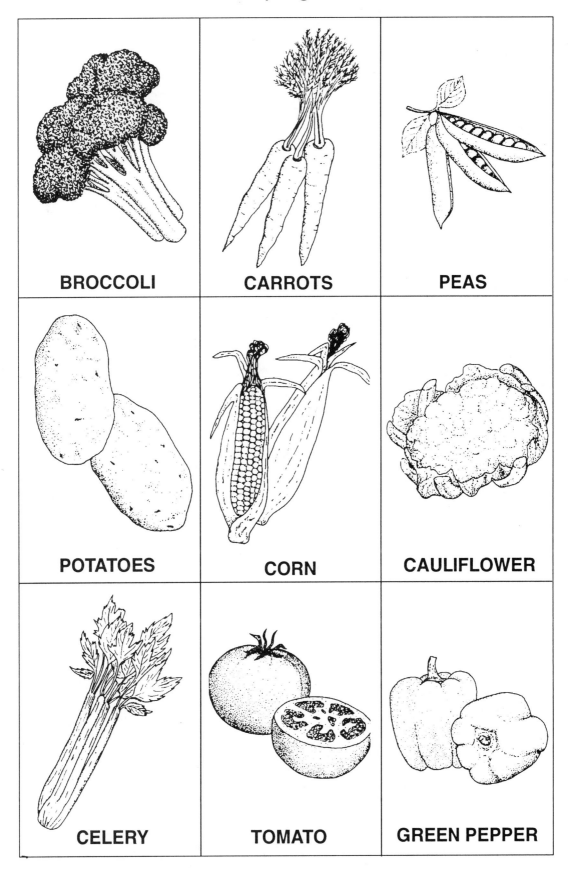

BREAD, CEREAL, RICE, AND PASTA Playing Cards (DN-30)

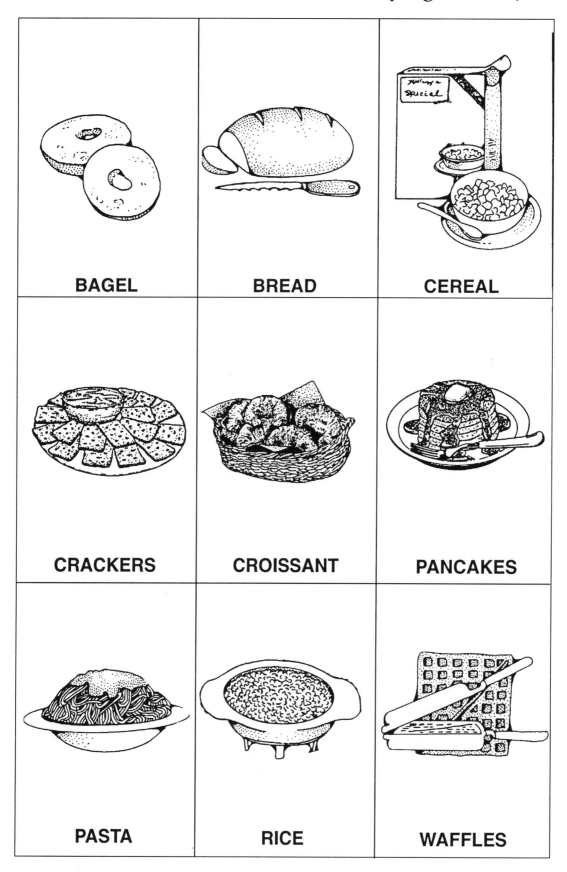

BAGEL	**BREAD**	**CEREAL**
CRACKERS	**CROISSANT**	**PANCAKES**
PASTA	**RICE**	**WAFFLES**

MEAT, POULTRY, FISH, DRY BEANS, EGGS, AND NUTS
Playing Cards (DN-31)

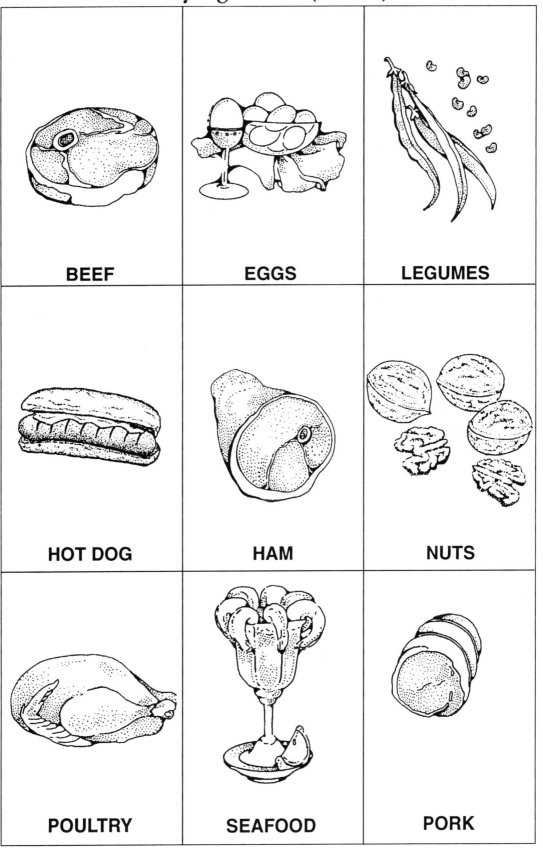

BEEF	**EGGS**	**LEGUMES**
HOT DOG	**HAM**	**NUTS**
POULTRY	**SEAFOOD**	**PORK**

FOOD GUIDE PYRAMID (DN-32)

DIRECTIONS: Place each food in its proper area on the food pyramid by drawing a line from the food to the correct area. The Agriculture Department unveiled the pyramid as the new shape for the ideal American diet in place of the old pie chart.

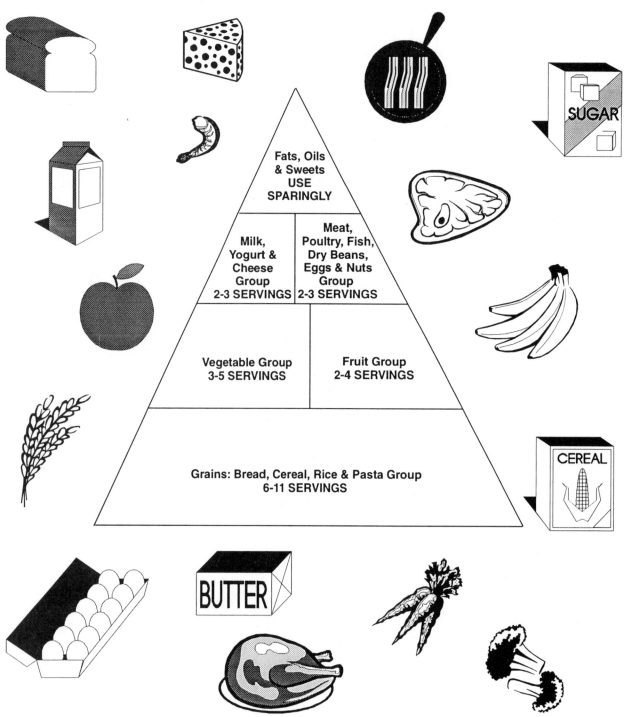

Fats, Oils
& Sweets
USE
SPARINGLY

Milk,
Yogurt &
Cheese
Group
2-3 SERVINGS

Meat,
Poultry, Fish,
Dry Beans,
Eggs & Nuts
Group
2-3 SERVINGS

Vegetable Group
3-5 SERVINGS

Fruit Group
2-4 SERVINGS

Grains: Bread, Cereal, Rice & Pasta Group
6-11 SERVINGS

SUGAR

CEREAL

BUTTER

©1993 by The Center for Applied Research in Education

U.S. RDA INFORMATION SHEET (DN-33)

Many nutrients on a food label are listed as a percentage of the U.S. Recommended Daily Allowances. The U.S. RDA are the amount of nutrients needed each day by most healthy people.

The following are U.S. RDA for these nutrients:

PROTEIN	45 g
VITAMIN A	5000 IU
VITAMIN C	60 mg
THIAMIN	1.5 mg
RIBOFLAVIN	1.7 mg
NIACIN	20 mg
CALCIUM	1000 mg
IRON	18 mg

DIRECTIONS: Look at the food label below and answer the questions.

TONS-O-BRAN CEREAL

PERCENTAGES OF U.S. RECOMMENDED DAILY ALLOWANCES

Protein	5 %
Vitamin A	25 %
Vitamin C	4 %
Thiamine	25 %
Riboflavin	25 %
Calcium	2 %
Iron	45 %
Vitamin D	10 %

How many bowls of cereal would you have to eat to meet the U.S. RDA for:

1. Vitamin A ?_____

2. Protein ?_____

3. Calcium ?_____

What would be a better way to meet the U.S. RDA? Explain.

ACTIVITY 8: PUT THE LABEL ON THE TABLE

Concept/ Description: The U.S. Food and Drug Administration requires certain information for every prepackaged food.

Objective: To look at various labels and determine the types of information required.

Materials: Empty boxes, cans, or bags of food
Food labels

Directions:
1. Have students bring in empty food containers and labels.

2. In groups of three or four, ask students to list the kinds of information their cartons contain. Write their answers on the board.

3. Refer to the U.S. RDA INFORMATION SHEET (DN-33) and the UNDERSTANDING FOOD LABELS sheet (DN-35) and explain the following:

   A. The U.S. F.D.A. requires that every prepackaged food is labeled with four kinds of information:
      - Name of product
      - Name and address of manufacturer
      - Weight of food without its container (net weight)
      - List of ingredients in descending weight order

   B. Many foods also list nutritional information based on the U.S. RDA.

   C. Detailed nutrition labels are only required by law on foods whose labels make a nutritional claim such as "Low Fat," "Low Cholesterol," "Enriched," etc. All other nutrition labelling is optional.

4. Discuss how some labels can be misleading. For example, using unusual serving sizes so consumers will have difficulty comparison shopping, or claiming that a product such as vegetable oil has "no cholesterol" when, in fact, cholesterol comes only from animal food sources.

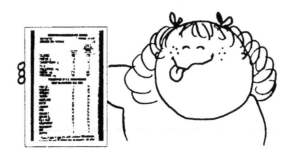

Name _____ **Date** _____

LABEL ABLE (DN-34)

DIRECTIONS: Refer to the Understanding Food Labels worksheet and answer the following
questions:

1. How many *total* ounces of Grain Grungies Cereal are in a box? _____

2. How many calories in a serving of Grain Grungies Cereal come from protein?_____

3. How many calories come from carbohydrates?_____

4. How many calories come from fat? _____

5. Name the four minerals that Grain Grungies Cereal lists in the U.S. RDA:

   _____

   _____

   _____

   _____

6. Is Grain Grungies Cereal considered a good fiber source? _____

7. Why or why not? _____

8. What ingredient in Grain Grungies Cereal is present in the largest amount?_____

   _____

9. How do you know that? _____

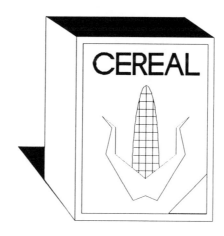

UNDERSTANDING FOOD LABELS (DN-35)

GRAIN GRUNGIES CEREAL

NUTRITION INFORMATION PER SERVING
SERVING SIZE...........1.3 OUNCE (3/4 CUP)
SERVINGS PER PACKAGE.....................11

CALORIES	130
PROTEIN	3 g
CARBOHYDRATE	28 g
FAT	2 g
CHOLESTEROL	0 mg
SODIUM	210 mg
POTASSIUM	100 mg

PERCENTAGE OF U.S. RECOMMENDED DAILY ALLOWANCES (U.S. RDA)

PROTEIN	4 %
VITAMIN A	25 %
VITAMIN C	25 %
THIAMIN	25 %
RIBOFLAVIN	25 %
NIACIN	25 %
CALCIUM	20 %
IRON	25 %
VITAMIN D	10 %
VITAMIN B 6	25 %
FOLIC ACID	25 %
PHOSPHORUS	15 %
MAGNESIUM	6 %
ZINC	4 %
COPPER	6 %

CARBOHYDRATE INFORMATION

DIETARY FIBER	2 g
COMPLEX CARBOHYDRATE	18 g

INGREDIENTS: CORN MEAL, WHEAT BRAN, SUGAR, WHOLE GRAIN BARLEY, WHOLE GRAIN ROLLED OATS, RICE, ~OWN SUGAR, ALMONDS, RAISINS, ~UTS, SALT, DRIED APPLES, ~AL AND NATURAL FLAVORS.

Serving size: There are no standard serving sizes. All the information is based on the serving size. In order to compare products make sure the serving sizes are the same.

Calories: These come from protein, carbohydrates and fats. It is now believed that more calories should come from carbohydrates and fewer from fats.

Protein: (in grams per serving) 1 gram of protein is equal to 4 calories.

Carbohydrates: (in grams) Some labels give a breakdown by type of carbohydrate: Complex Fiber and Sucrose or Other Sugars. 1 gram carbohydrate = 4 calories and 4 grams sucrose = 1 teaspoon of table sugar.

Fats: (in grams) 1 gram fat = 9 calories. Five grams of fat is equal to 1 teaspoon of oil, butter, or margarine.

Cholesterol: This listing is required only if the manufacturer makes a cholesterol claim. Some high-cholesterol foods, like meat, eggs, and cheese, often have no labels. And some foods that boast of "no cholesterol" may be high in saturated fat, which can raise the blood cholesterol more than cholesterol from food.

Sodium: (in milligrams) Experts recommend we limit this to 3000 milligrams per day. One teaspoon of salt has 2,300 mg of sodium.

U.S. Recommended Daily Allowances: Labels must include RDAs for protein, at least five vitamins, and two minerals (calcium and iron).

Fiber: Cereals, vegetables, fruits and nuts contain fiber. Foods with 3 grams or more are good fiber sources.

Ingredients listing: This shows contents of the product in order of amount by weight.

©1993 by The Center for Applied Research in Education

UNIT PRICING AND OPEN DATING (DN-36)

Unit pricing shows a person how much different sizes of the same product cost per unit. For example, suppose that you wanted to buy one can of Puppy Treat Dog Food. One 9-ounce can costs 99 cents. The unit price per ounce is, therefore, 11 cents. A 12-ounce can of the same brand is $1.04. The unit price is approximately 8.7 cents. You would save over 3 cents per ounce if you bought the larger can. (Note: Keep in mind that if you purchase the larger, better-priced item, you should be able to use the extra ounces of the product. If they would go to waste, it may not be the better buy.) Unit price labels are found on grocery store shelves with the calculations already done for the shopper. This allows you to compare the prices of different brands.

　　Open dating provides a date on a product that tells you when it should be removed from the shelves, when it should be used by, or when it was packaged.

DIRECTIONS: On the survey form below, select three food items, go to the grocery store, and do unit pricing for different brands of each item. Place an asterisk (*) next to the best buy for each item. Report your findings back to the class.

©1993 by The Center for Applied Research in Education

FOOD ITEM	SIZE	TOTAL PRICE	UNIT PRICE
ITEM #1:			
1			
2			
3			
4			
5			
ITEM #2:			
1			
2			
3			
4			
5			
ITEM #3:			
1			
2			
3			
4			
5			

FOOD SAFETY

- **Food Additives**

- **Safety Tips**

ACTIVITY 9: FOOD INSPECTOR

Concept/ Description: The growing concern about food safety focuses on the use and possible dangers of pesticides and food additives.

Objective: To have students research topics dealing with food safety and report the findings back to the class.

Materials: Reference books
Consumer magazines
Health newsletter
Newspaper articles
Paper
Pens or pencils

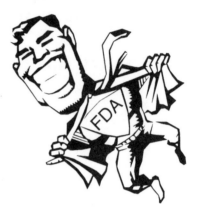

Directions:

1. Assign groups of three to four one of the following topics:

Food Additives:	Red Dye #2
Colorings	DDT
Flavorings	Cyanide in Grapes
Stabilizers	Alar in Apples
Preservatives	Sulfites
Organic Farming	Antibiotics in Meats
U.S. FDA	Pesticides
EPA	Salmonella
USDA	Botulism
GRAS	The Delaney Clause

2. Each topic above is somehow related to food safety, be it an organization designed to insure food safety, a food additive, a recent food safety controversy, a foodborne illness, or food safety legislation.

3. Ask each group to research the topic to determine how and why it relates to food safety.

4. Groups should prepare a 2- to 3-minute oral report on their assigned topic and present it to the class.

5. As the groups are giving the report, prepare a quiz on the information presented; or, allow each group to submit two questions from their talk and put the questions together for a quiz.

WHAT IS THAT STUFF? (DN-37)

DIRECTIONS: Listed below are some common types of additives, what they do, and examples of each. Do you recognize any of these names? Look on the labels of some of your favorite foods. Which additives are in the foods? Why are they there?

CATEGORY	WHAT IT DOES	EXAMPLES
NUTRIENTS	Added to make food more nutritious or to replace nutrients lost in processing	ascorbic acid, beta carotene, iodine, iron, niacinamide, potassium idodide, riboflavin, thiamin, vitamins A, C, D, E
PRESERVATIVES	Prevent foods from spoiling due to bacteria, fungi, molds, and yeast; extend shelf-life of food; protect natural flavor and color of food	ascorbic acid, benzoic acid, butylparaben, calcium lactate, calcium propionate, calcium sorbate, citric acid, heptylparaben, lactic acid, methylparaben, potassium propionate, potassium sorbate, propionic acid, propylparaben, sodium benzoate, sodium diacetate, sodium erythorbate, sodium nitrate, sodium nitrite, sodium propionate, sodium sorbate, sorbic acid
ANTIOXIDANTS	Slow down and prevent rancidity or browning due to enzyme activity	ascorbic acid, BHA, BHT, citric acid, EDTA, propyl gallate, TBHQ, vitamin E
EMULSIFIERS	Help prevent separation of liquids; help improve texture and consistency	carrageenan, diglycerides, dioctyl sodium sulfosccinate, lecithin, monoglycerides, polysorbates, sorbitan monostearate
STABILIZERS, THICKENERS, TEXTURIZERS	Give food body, improve texture or consistency; stabilize emulsions; affect food texture	ammonium alginate, arabinogalactan, carob bean gum, calcium alginate, carrageenan, cellulose, gelatin, guar gum, gum arabic, gum ghatti, karaya gum, larch gum, locust bean gum, mannitol, modified food starch, pectin, potassium alginate, propylene glycol, sodium alginate, sodium calcium alginate, tragacanth gum
LEAVENING AGENTS	Affect cooking results of texture and volume	calcium phosphate, sodium aluminum sulfate, sodium bicarbonate
pH CONTROL AGENTS	Change and/or maintain acidity or alkalinity of food	acetic acid, adipic acid, citric acid, lactic acid, phosphates, phosphoric acid, sodium acetate, sodium citrate, tartaric acid
HUMECTANTS	Cause food to retain moisture	glycerine, glycerol monostearate, propylene glycol, sorbitol
MATURING AND BLEACHING AGENTS	Accelerate the food aging process, improve the quality of baking	acetone peroxide, azodicarbonamide, benzoyl peroxide, calcium bromate, hydrogen peroxide, potassium bromate, sodium stearyl fumarate
ANTI-CAKING AGENTS	Prevent caking, lumping, or clustering of powdered or crystalline substances	cornstarch

ADDITIVES OR PRESERVATIVES? (DN-38)

DIRECTIONS: If the boldface term in each sentence is correct, leave it as is. If it is **not** correct, cross it out and write the correct term in the space provided. All categories of additives are in the box below:

nutrients   leavening agents
preservatives   pH control agents
antioxidants   emulsifiers
humectants   stabilizers
anti-caking agents   maturing and bleaching agents

1. **Nutrients** are substances added to food to make it more nutritious, such as vitamins or minerals. _____

2. **Texturizers**, such as citric acid and sorbic acid, help prevent food spoilage from microorganisms. _____

3. **Emulsifiers** delay and prevent rancidity or enzymatic browning. Examples are BHA and BHT. _____

4. **Humectants** like sorbitol and glycerine cause foods to retain moisture. _____

5. **Anti-caking agents** affect cooking texture and volume. _____

6. **Leavening agents** change and/or maintain acidity or alkalinity. _____

7. Polysorbates and diglycerides are **preservatives** that help to keep liquids from separating. _____

8. **Stabilizers** improve texture, consistency, and body. _____

9. **Maturing and bleaching agents** improve baking qualities and accelerate the food aging process. _____

10. **Humectants** prevent caking and lumping. _____

FOOD SAFETY RULES (DN-39)

Listed below are some ways to protect yourself against foodborne illness:

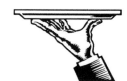

1. Wash your hands before working with food.

2. Discard food that you suspect is spoiled. Trust your suspicions.

3. Cook foods such as meats and poultry at high temperatures to prevent bacteria growth.

4. Never leave meat, poultry, or fish at room temperature to thaw. To prevent growth of bacteria, allow food to thaw in the refrigerator.

5. Use soap and hot water to scrub cutting boards especially after using them to prepare meat or poultry. If not cleaned properly, bacteria can contaminate the board and it could be spread to other foods.

6. Don't buy damaged or bulging packaged or canned goods.

7. Rinse can tops with hot water before opening.

8. Check the expiration date on perishable foods.

9. Thoroughly rinse and scrub all fruits and vegetables to wash off any pesticides and remove the outer leaves of leafy vegetables for the same reason.

10. Buy lean meats and trim off any visible fat, because pesticide residues may be stored in animal fat.

EATING HEALTHY

- Balanced Diets

- Dietary Concerns

- Snacking

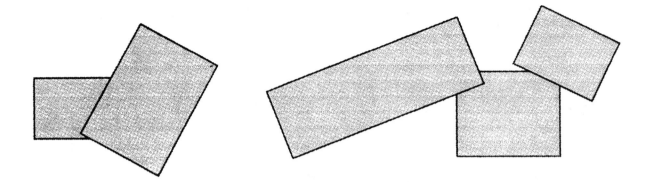

FOOD CARDS

The following food cards are designed to be used in a variety of ways. There are many games and activities provided that make use of the cards, and you are encouraged to create and develop ideas of your own.

The cards can be given to groups for ranking from least to most according to sodium, calories, fat, carbohydrates, cholesterol, or protein. They can also be used as a reference or as a discussion starter.

The best way to save them for future use is to laminate them and cut them or to cut them and paste them onto index cards. They are placed in the appropriate food groups for your convenience.

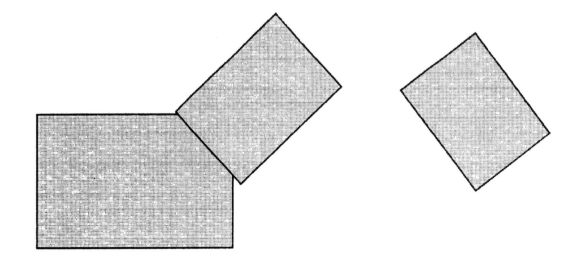

BREAD, CEREAL, RICE, AND PASTA Cards (DN-40)

RYE BREAD (1 slice)

Calories	65
Protein	2 g
Carbohydrate	12 g
Fat	1 g
Cholesterol	0 mg
Sodium	175 mg

EGG NOODLES (1/2 cup)

Calories	106
Protein	4 g
Carbohydrate	20 g
Fat	1 g
Cholesterol	26 mg
Sodium	5 mg

ENGLISH MUFFIN (1/2 muffin)

Calories	70
Protein	3 g
Carbohydrate	14 g
Fat	1 g
Cholesterol	0 mg
Sodium	189 mg

WHITE BREAD (1 slice)

Calories	65
Protein	2 g
Carbohydrate	12 g
Fat	1 g
Cholesterol	0 mg
Sodium	129 mg

RICE (White, long-grain, cooked, 1/2 cup)

Calories	131
Protein	3 g
Carbohydrate	28 g
Fat	0 g
Cholesterol	0 mg
Sodium	2 mg

OATMEAL (Instant, cooked, 1/2 cup)

Calories	73
Protein	3 g
Carbohydrate	13 g
Fat	1 g
Cholesterol	NA
Sodium	1 mg

WHEAT BREAD (1 slice)

Calories	70
Protein	3 g
Carbohydrate	13 g
Fat	1 g
Cholesterol	0 mg
Sodium	180 mg

CORN FLAKES (1 ounce)

Calories	110
Protein	2 g
Carbohydrate	24 g
Fat	0 g
Cholesterol	NA
Sodium	351 mg

MILK, YOGURT, AND CHEESE Cards (DN-41)

PLAIN YOGURT, Nonfat (1 cup)

Calories	127
Protein	13 g
Carbohydrate	17 g
Fat	0 g
Cholesterol	4 mg
Sodium	174 mg

BUTTER (1 teaspoon)

Calories	34
Protein	0 g
Carbohydrate	0 g
Fat	4 g
Cholesterol	10 mg
Sodium	39 mg

PARMESAN CHEESE (1 tablespoon)

Calories	23
Protein	2 g
Carbohydrate	0 g
Fat	2 g
Cholesterol	4 mg
Sodium	93 mg

AMERICAN CHEESE (1 ounce)

Calories	106
Protein	6 g
Carbohydrate	0 g
Fat	9 g
Cholesterol	27 mg
Sodium	406 mg

2% LOWFAT COTTAGE CHEESE (1/2 cup)

Calories	102
Protein	16 g
Carbohydrate	3 g
Fat	5 g
Cholesterol	16 mg
Sodium	425 mg

WHOLE MILK (1 cup)

Calories	150
Protein	8 g
Carbohydrate	11 g
Fat	8 g
Cholesterol	33 mg
Sodium	120 mg

SOFT ICE CREAM (1/2 cup)

Calories	189
Protein	4 g
Carbohydrate	19 g
Fat	11 g
Cholesterol	77 mg
Sodium	77 mg

SWISS CHEESE (1 ounce)

Calories	107
Protein	8 g
Carbohydrate	1 g
Fat	8 g
Cholesterol	26 mg
Sodium	74 mg

FRUIT Cards (DN-42)

ORANGE (1 medium)

Calories	65
Protein	1 g
Carbohydrate	15 g
Fat	0 g
Cholesterol	0 mg
Sodium	0 mg

STRAWBERRIES (1/2 cup)

Calories	24
Protein	0 g
Carbohydrate	5 g
Fat	0 g
Cholesterol	0 mg
Sodium	1 mg

APPLE (1 medium)

Calories	80
Protein	0 g
Carbohydrate	21 g
Fat	0 g
Cholesterol	0 g
Sodium	1 mg

GRAPES (1/2 cup)

Calories	30
Protein	0 g
Carbohydrate	8 g
Fat	0 g
Cholesterol	0 mg
Sodium	1 mg

CANNED PEARS (1/2 cup in juice)

Calories	62
Protein	0 g
Carbohydrate	16 g
Fat	0 g
Cholesterol	0 mg
Sodium	5 mg

WATERMELON (1/2 cup)

Calories	25
Protein	0 g
Carbohydrate	6 g
Fat	0 g
Cholesterol	0 mg
Sodium	2 mg

BANANA (1 medium)

Calories	105
Protein	1 g
Carbohydrate	27 g
Fat	1 g
Cholesterol	0 mg
Sodium	1 mg

GRAPEFRUIT (1/2 medium)

Calories	40
Protein	1 g
Carbohydrate	10 g
Fat	0 g
Cholesterol	0 mg
Sodium	0 mg

FATS, OILS, AND SWEETS Cards (DN-43)

GLAZED DOUGHNUT

Calories	235
Protein	4 g
Carbohydrate	26 g
Fat	13 g
Cholesterol	21 mg
Sodium	222 mg

CHOCOLATE CANDY BAR (1 ounce)

Calories	145
Protein	2 g
Carbohydrate	16 g
Fat	9 g
Cholesterol	6 mg
Sodium	23 mg

PEANUT BUTTER (2 tablespoons)

Calories	188
Protein	8 g
Carbohydrate	7 g
Fat	16 g
Cholesterol	7 0 mg
Sodium	153 mg

JELLY (1 teaspoon)

Calories	17
Protein	0 g
Carbohydrate	4 g
Fat	0 g
Cholesterol	0 mg
Sodium	2 mg

SOFT DRINK (12 fluid ounces)

Calories	151
Protein	0 g
Carbohydrate	39 g
Fat	0 g
Cholesterol	0 mg
Sodium	14 mg

CHOCOLATE CAKE (1/16 of 9-inch cake)

Calories	235
Protein	3 g
Carbohydrate	40 g
Fat	8 g
Cholesterol	37 mg
Sodium	181 mg

BACON (3 slices)

Calories	109
Protein	6 g
Carbohydrate	0 g
Fat	9 g
Cholesterol	16 mg
Sodium	303 mg

POTATO CHIPS (1 ounce)

Calories	148
Protein	2 g
Carbohydrate	15 g
Fat	10 g
Cholesterol	0 mg
Sodium	133 mg

VEGETABLE Cards (DN-44)

BROCCOLI (Fresh, cooked, 1/2 cup)

Calories	23
Protein	2 g
Carbohydrate	4 g
Fat	0 g
Cholesterol	0 mg
Sodium	8 mg

GREEN BEANS (Fresh, cooked, 1/2 cup)

Calories	22
Protein	1 g
Carbohydrate	5 g
Fat	0 g
Cholesterol	0 mg
Sodium	2 mg

CELERY (1 stalk)

Calories	6
Protein	0 g
Carbohydrate	1 g
Fat	0 g
Cholesterol	0 mg
Sodium	35 mg

BAKED POTATO (Flesh and skin, 1 large)

Calories	220
Protein	5 g
Carbohydrate	51 g
Fat	0 g
Cholesterol	0 mg
Sodium	16 mg

CARROTS (Fresh, cooked, 1/2 cup)

Calories	35
Protein	1 g
Carbohydrate	8 g
Fat	0 g
Cholesterol	0 mg
Sodium	25 mg

CORN (Frozen, cooked, 1/2 cup)

Calories	67
Protein	2 g
Carbohydrate	17 g
Fat	0 g
Cholesterol	0 mg
Sodium	4 mg

CAULIFLOWER (Fresh, cooked, 1/2 cup)

Calories	15
Protein	1 g
Carbohydrate	3 g
Fat	0 g
Cholesterol	0 mg
Sodium	4 mg

GREEN PEAS (Frozen, cooked, 1/2 cup)

Calories	63
Protein	4 g
Carbohydrate	11 g
Fat	0 g
Cholesterol	0 mg
Sodium	70 mg

MEAT, POULTRY, FISH, DRY BEANS, EGGS, AND NUTS Cards (DN-45)

HARD-COOKED EGG (1 egg)

Calories	79
Protein	6 g
Carbohydrate	0 g
Fat	6 g
Cholesterol	274 mg
Sodium	69 mg

SIRLOIN STEAK (3 ounces)

Calories	180
Protein	26 g
Carbohydrate	0 g
Fat	8 g
Cholesterol	76 mg
Sodium	56 mg

SHRIMP (Boiled, 3 ounces)

Calories	84
Protein	18 g
Carbohydrate	0 g
Fat	1 g
Cholesterol	166 mg
Sodium	190 mg

TUNA IN WATER (Canned, 3 ounces)

Calories	116
Protein	23 g
Carbohydrate	0 g
Fat	2 g
Cholesterol	35 mg
Sodium	376 mg

BEEF HOT DOG (2 ounces)

Calories	184
Protein	6 g
Carbohydrate	1 g
Fat	17 g
Cholesterol	27 mg
Sodium	584 mg

NAVY BEANS (Canned, 1/2 cup)

Calories	148
Protein	10 g
Carbohydrate	27 g
Fat	1 g
Cholesterol	0 mg
Sodium	587 mg

PORK CHOP (Broiled, 3 ounces)

Calories	219
Protein	25 g
Carbohydrate	0 g
Fat	13 g
Cholesterol	80 mg
Sodium	57 mg

HAM (11% fat, 3 ounces)

Calories	156
Protein	15 g
Carbohydrate	3 g
Fat	9 g
Cholesterol	48 mg
Sodium	1119 mg

LET'S DO LUNCH! (DN-46)

DIRECTIONS: Look at the lunch below. Use the Food Cards (DN-40 to DN-45) to answer the questions in the box. Is this a nutritious lunch? Why or why not?

1 slice of white bread + **1 slice of white bread** + **2 tbsp. of peanut butter** +

2 tsp. of jelly + **1 medium apple** + **1 cup of whole milk** =

Total number of calories _____

Total grams of fat _____

Total milligrams of cholesterol _____

Total milligrams of sodium _____

Total grams of protein _____

Total grams of carbohydrates _____

Name _____   Date _____

FOOD CARDS QUESTIONNAIRE (DN-47)

DIRECTIONS: Refer to the FOOD CARDS (DN-40 to DN-45) and answer the following questions:

1. Which **group** of foods is highest in sodium? _____

2. Which food is highest in sodium? _____

3. Which **group** of foods is lowest in carbohydrates? _____

4. Which **three groups** are very low in cholesterol? _____

                                   _____

                                     _____

5. Which food is highest in cholesterol? _____

6. Which food is lowest in calories? _____

7. Which **two foods** are highest in calories?_____

                                     _____

8. Which vegetable is highest in carbohydrates? _____

9. Which food from the meat group has the most fat? _____

                     How much? _____

10. Which food from the grains group is highest in sodium? _____

                     Lowest? _____

ACTIVITY 10: THE PRESSURE'S ON!

**Concept/
Description:** Foods vary in the amount of sodium, cholesterol, and fat that they contain. Limiting the amount of these substances in the diet can help reduce the risk of heart disease.

Objective: To be the player with the least amount of sodium, cholesterol, or fat when the food cards are totalled.

Materials: Food Cards (DN-40 to DN-45)
The Pressure's On! Scorecard
Pens or pencils

Directions: 1. Prior to class, photocopy one set of Food Cards for each group of six. Then photocopy one The Pressure's On! Scorecard for each person.

2. Divide the class into groups of six and give each group a set of Food Cards, which have been cut apart and shuffled. Turn the cards face down on the desk or playing surface.

3. One at a time, in turn, each player draws a card, turns it face up and announces the food and the amount of sodium. That person then records the amount of sodium on their score card under the sodium column. Continue choosing and recording until all forty-eight cards have been selected.

4. Each player adds up the total amount of sodium on their cards and the player with the fewest milligrams is the winner.

5. Shuffle the cards and play again, but for this round, count total milligrams of cholesterol. Once again, the lowest amount wins.

6. Shuffle and play round three counting grams of fat. Again, the lowest amount of fat is the winner.

7. Discuss the effects large amounts of sodium, cholesterol, and fat have on health.

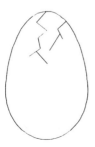 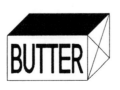 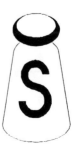

Name _____ **Date** _____

THE PRESSURE'S ON! Scorecard (DN-48)

SODIUM	CHOLESTEROL	FAT
TOTAL_____ mg	TOTAL_____ mg	TOTAL_____ g
TOTAL_____ mg	TOTAL_____ mg	TOTAL_____ g
TOTAL_____ mg	TOTAL_____ mg	TOTAL_____ g

©1993 by The Center for Applied Research in Education

ACTIVITY 11: HOSPITAL FOOD

Concept/ Description: People with high blood pressure, high cholesterol, or heart disease may require modified diets.

Objective: To develop a balanced diet for each "patient" based on his or her particular needs.

Materials: Food Cards (DN-40 to DN-45)
Patient List and Menu Planner (DN-49)

Directions:
1. Divide the class into groups of four to six.
2. Give each group a set of Food Cards and a Patient List and Menu Planner.
3. Ask the groups to devise a balanced breakfast, lunch, and dinner for each patient using the food on the food cards. The groups should be prepared to explain their choices.
4. Have each group explain their menu for any one patient to the class.
5. Discuss.

"I just remembered...I'm really not THAT hungry!!"

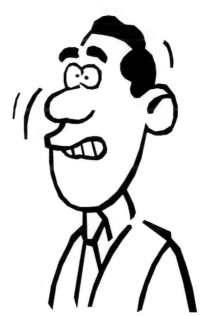

MENU
1. **Cow's tongue**
2. **Liver souffle**
3. **Sweetbreads**
4. **Ostrich casserole**
5. **Pig's knuckles**

PATIENT LIST AND MENU PLANNER (DN-49)

DIRECTIONS: Refer to the food cards to develop a balanced breakfast, lunch, and dinner for each of the hospital "patients" described below. Be sure to keep the patient's particular needs in mind when developing the day's menu.

Mr. Smith
50-year-old male
High Blood Pressure
Ulcer

Breakfast:

Lunch:

Dinner:

Ms. Rodgers
48-year-old female
Obese
High Cholesterol
Heart Disease

Breakfast:

Lunch:

Dinner:

Shannon Jackson
10-year-old female
Had tonsils out
Has a sore throat

Breakfast:

Lunch:

Dinner:

Mr. Brown
65-year-old male
Has no teeth
Heart Disease

Breakfast:

Lunch:

Dinner:

THE AMERICAN DIET (DN-50)

DIRECTIONS: The graph below compares the average American diet with a diet recommended by many leading nutrition experts. Use the graph to answer the questions.

IN PERCENTAGES

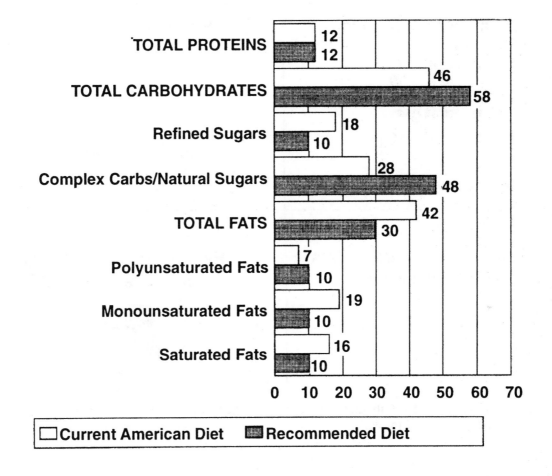

©1993 by The Center for Applied Research in Education

1. What percentage of the American diet is made up of saturated fats?_____
2. What is recommended?_____
3. What percentage of the American diet is made up of all fats?_____
4. What is recommended?_____
5. What category remains the same for the current and recommended diets?_____
6. By how much does the recommended diet suggest that Americans cut their use of refined sugars?_____
7. By how much does the recommended diet suggest Americans increase complex carbohydrate consumption?_____

DIETARY GUIDELINES FOR AMERICANS (DN-51)

Studies have shown that the average American eats too much fat, sugar, and sodium and too little fiber. Obesity is a health concern that has been linked to problems such as high blood pressure, heart disease, and cancer. To encourage people to improve their eating habits, the U.S. Government developed Dietary Guidelines for Americans. Here are some of the suggestions:

Eat a variety of foods.

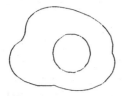

Select foods each day from each food group.

Maintain an ideal weight.

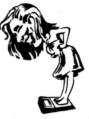

Exercise and choose foods that provide high nutrition in relation to calories.

Limit intake of saturated fats and cholesterol.

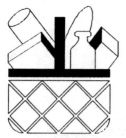

Choose lean meats, poultry, fish. Limit eggs, butter, and fried foods.

Eat foods with an adequate supply of starch and fiber

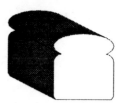

Eat whole-grain breads and cereals, fruits, vegetables, and legumes.

Avoid too much sugar.

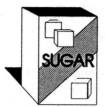

Limit intake of sweet snacks, candy, and soft drinks. Eat fresh fruits instead.

Limit intake of sodium.

Reduce salt in cooking and at the table. Limit salty snacks, pickled foods, cured meats, and canned soups.

ACTIVITY 12: SNACK MANIAC

Concept/ Description: Many snacks are high in sugar, fat, salt, and calories but have little nutritive value.

Objective: To make a visual display of nutritious and non-nutritious snacks.

Materials: Magazine pictures of food
Food labels
Scissors
Glue or paste
Markers, colored pens or colored pencils
Snack Maniac worksheet (DN-52, 53)

Directions:
1. On the board, make a list of snacks that students enjoy eating. Ask if the snacks are nutritious. Why or why not? Do the snacks contain a lot of fat, salt, sugar, or calories?

2. Next, discuss snacks that would be nutritious and why.

3. Give each student both of the Snack Maniac worksheets and have them draw or cut out and paste pictures that would fit the two headings. They should place their pictures in the two stomachs. Suggestions for each heading are written below.

4. Display the best papers.

EAT MORE OF THESE SNACKS:
Whole-grain muffins
Whole-grain crackers
Frozen yogurt
Sherbet
Ice milk
Skim milk
Unsalted popcorn
Unsalted nuts
Whole-grain cereals
Fresh vegetables
Dried fruits
Fresh fruits

EAT FEWER OF THESE SNACKS:
Canned fruits
Pudding
Cakes
Cookies
Doughnuts
Pastries
Whole milk
Ice cream
Potato chips
Pretzels
Corn chips
Fried foods
Candy
Chocolate

SNACK MANIAC (DN-52)

EAT MORE OF THESE SNACKS:

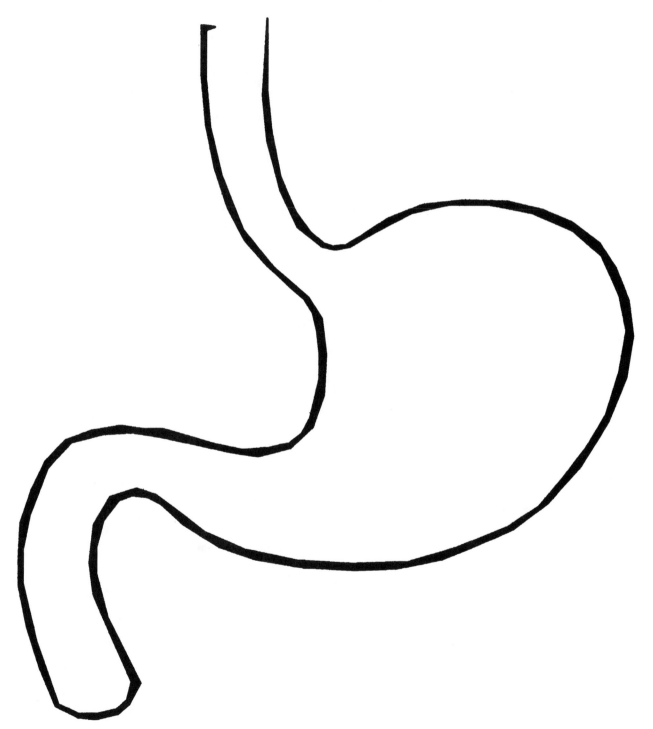

SNACK MANIAC (DN-53)

EAT FEWER OF THESE SNACKS:

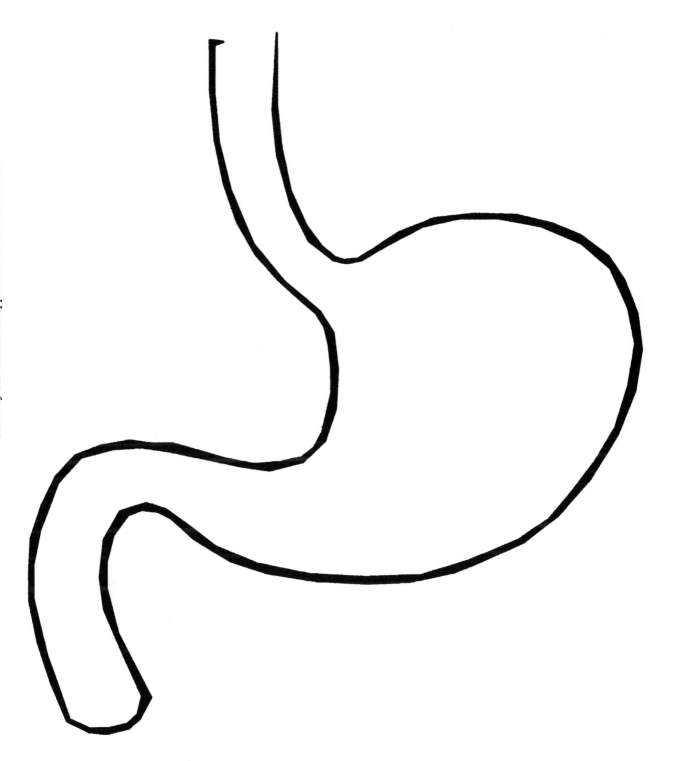

ACTIVITY 13: SNACK ATTACK

Concept/
Description: Many snacks are high in salt, sugar, fat, and calories and have little nutritive value.

Objective: To determine whether the snacks students eat are nutritious.

Materials: Snack Attack Chart (DN-54)
Pens or pencils
Scrap paper

Directions:
1. Have each student take out a piece of scrap paper and a pen or pencil.
2. Ask students to list all of the snack foods they like to eat.
3. When they are finished, hand each student a Snack Attack Chart.
4. Have students copy all the snacks that they listed onto the chart under the proper food group.
5. Survey the class to determine which food group most of the snacks fall into.
6. Ask if students think their snack choices are nutritious.
7. As a group, list nutritious choices for snacks. Write the ideas on the board.

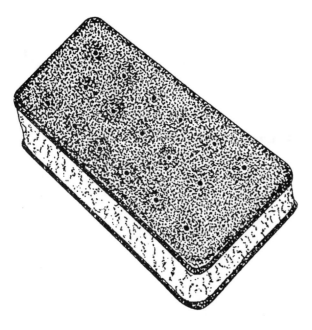 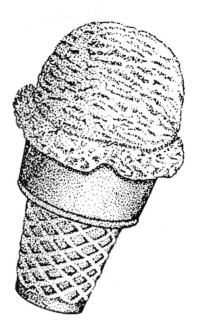

Name _____ **Date** _____

SNACK ATTACK Chart (DN-54)

DIRECTIONS: Write all the snacks you listed on the scrap paper on this sheet in the proper food group.

MILK GROUP

FRUIT GROUP

MEAT GROUP

VEGETABLE GROUP

GRAINS GROUP

FATS, OILS, SWEETS GROUP

INVISIBLE SUGAR (DN-55)

The average American consumes about 120 pounds of sugar each year, nearly 1/3 of a pound per day. Most of the sugar is from foods prepared outside of the home and is "invisible" because we don't normally associate it with the food. The body needs sugar obtained from carbohydrates found naturally in fruits, vegetables, and grains. Refined sugar, or table sugar, provides energy but no proteins, fats, vitamins, or fiber. Sugar is a carbohydrate and is called by many different names, such as:

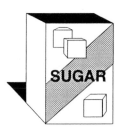

SUCROSE	table sugar
LACTOSE	milk sugar
GLUCOSE	blood sugar
FRUCTOSE	fruit sugar
DEXTROSE	fruit sugar
MALTOSE	starch sugar
GALACTOSE	part of milk sugar

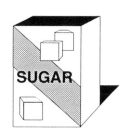

DIRECTIONS: Check the labels of ten prepared foods in your home and write down the product and type of sugar listed. Note: Sugar may be listed as sugar, corn syrup, or one of the names listed above.

Product	Type of Sugar Listed
Instant Pudding	Sugar, dextrose (from corn)

©1993 by The Center for Applied Research in Education

FACTORS AFFECTING DIET

- General

- Personal Taste

- Emotions

- Advertising

CHOCOLATE-COVERED ANTS, ANYONE? (DN-56)

DIRECTIONS: Many factors influence our eating habits. Write down some foods that you eat for each reason listed below.

Family Customs:

Ethnic Background:

Economics:

Geography and Climate:

Availability:

Convenience:

Personal Taste:

ACTIVITY 14: DARE TO COMPARE

Concept/ Description: Processed foods are convenient but often lack many features of homemade food.

Objective: To compare a homemade food with a store-bought food.

Materials: Foods to be compared
Taste Test Sheet (DN-57)
Pens or pencils

Directions:
1. If possible, arrange to prepare a homemade item, such as a pie or cake, in conjunction with your home economics department. Get a copy of the recipe to distribute to the class.
2. If this is not possible, have a student make the item for extra credit or make it yourself and bring it to class.
3. Purchase a similar product, such as a frozen pie or cake.
4. Give students samples of each and have them rate each on the Taste Test Sheet. Note: Be sure to check if any students have food allergies or are unable to eat the food for any reason.
5. Discuss the results of the taste test and determine which food is preferable.

Variations:
1. Conduct a taste test with the faculty and compile the results.
2. Have students determine what foods they wish to compare.
3. Give extra credit for a family taste test project.

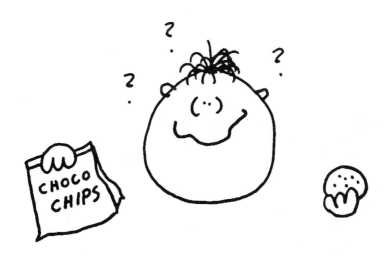

TASTE TEST SHEET (DN-57)

FOOD_____

	Homemade				Store-Bought			
CALORIES PER SERVING								
SODIUM PER SERVING								
COST PER SERVING								
TASTE	1	2	3	4	1	2	3	4
TEXTURE	1	2	3	4	1	2	3	4
APPEARANCE	1	2	3	4	1	2	3	4
CONVENIENCE	1	2	3	4	1	2	3	4
COLOR	1	2	3	4	1	2	3	4
OVERALL RATING	1	2	3	4	1	2	3	4

RATING SCALE: 1 = Excellent
2 = Good
3 = Fair
4 = Poor

VARIETY IS THE SPICE OF LIFE (DN-58)

DIRECTIONS: For each food group, write down some of the foods you enjoy. Compare your list to a classmate's. Are your tastes similar?

Food Group	Foods You Enjoy
Fats, Oils, Sweets	
Milk, Yogurt, Cheese	
Meat, Poultry, Fish, Dry Beans, Eggs, Nuts	
Fruit	
Vegetables	
Bread, Cereal, Rice, Pasta	

EATING AND EMOTIONS (DN-59)

Hunger, according to scientists, is physiological, a sensation that occurs when the blood sugar begins to drop and the stomach contracts. But we are all aware that many people eat for emotional reasons as well. Try the quiz below to give you some idea of how well attuned you are to your own habits and how your emotions influence your eating habits.

DIRECTIONS: Use the following guidelines to give yourself a score of 0–8 for each item:

8 **Very often**—almost every other day
6 **Often**—one to three times a week
4 **Occasionally**—two to three times a month
2 **Rarely**—once every month to three months
0 **Never**

1. I eat foods that I know aren't nutritious. _____
2. I eat meals or heavy snacks after 7 at night. _____
3. I'm afraid I'll gain weight. _____
4. I eat when I'm not hungry. _____
5. I eat foods my parents don't want me to eat. _____
6. I'm self-conscious about how I look. _____
7. When I'm bored or depressed, I eat a lot. _____
8. I go on eating binges. _____
9. I eat until I'm uncomfortable. _____
10. I hide foods or sneak them. _____
11. I eat because I feel "who cares"? _____
12. I drink alcoholic beverages. _____
13. I have uncontrollable urges of hunger. _____
14. Feelings of anger or hostility overwhelm me. _____
15. I indulge in sweets. _____
16. I eat when I'm tired or overtired. _____
17. I like to eat alone. _____
18. I use appetite suppressants. _____
19. My parents made sweets available or used them for rewards. _____
20. I eat and run. _____
21. I don't have respect for myself and my body. _____
22. I feel rushed or hurried. _____
23. I have a snack or meal an hour before I go to bed. _____
24. I crave sweet foods. _____
25. When I eat with other people, I feel self-conscious. _____
26. I gulp my food. _____
27. I wish I looked like someone else. _____
28. I eat or drink in secret. _____
29. I feel as if I'm in the middle of a struggle. _____
30. I eat when I can't sleep. _____

Name _____ Date _____

SCORING FOR EATING AND EMOTIONS (DN-60)

What your score means:

    120 and below: Good relationship with your body; sensitive to physical needs.
         120-160: Average range for normally healthy people.
         161-190: Eating is based too much on emotional needs
   191 and above: Excessive emotional interference in eating habits.

     When emotions lead to poor nutritional habits, it can affect the normal functioning of the body. This, in turn, can make us feel listless. Bingeing, gorging, eating at the wrong time, or constant snacking can result in bloating and eventually obesity. Eating too fast or too much can interfere with the digestive system's ability to use nutrients properly.

ANSWER THE FOLLOWING QUESTIONS:

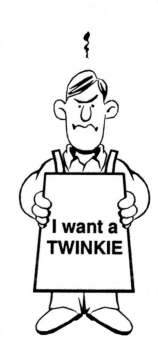

1. Into which category does your score place you?

2. Are you happy or unhappy with your eating habits? Explain.

3. What can you do to improve your eating habits? (List at least three suggestions.)

ACTIVITY 15: SENSE APPEAL

Concept/Description: Advertising is a powerful influence on our food choices.

Objective: To list the types of food commercials shown on television in a given period of time and to plot the results on a pie chart.

Materials: Food Ads Checklist (DN-61)
Food Ads Pie Chart (DN-62)
TV Sign-Up Sheet (DN-63)
Stopwatch or watch with second hand

Directions:
1. Give each student a Food Ads Checklist and a Food Ads Pie Chart.

2. Have students sign-up on the TV Sign-Up Sheet to watch television for 1 hour.

3. During the hour, students are to watch for food advertisements. On the Food Ads Checklist, write the name of the product advertised and the length of time the ad is aired.

4. Bring the results back to class.

5. Explain to the class how to take their results and make a pie graph:

   a. Add the total commercial time devoted to food.

   b. Figure the percentage of air time devoted to each category by dividing the total air time into the amount of time for each category. For example, if there were 10 total minutes of advertising of food products and 5 minutes were devoted to soft drinks and sugary snacks, then the percentage of time was 5/10 or 50 percent. If another 2 minutes were devoted to milk, cheese, and yogurt, the percentage would be 2/10 or 20 percent.

   c. Place the percentages on the pie chart, color code, and label as shown in the example.

Soft drinks, sugars 50.0%
Fruits, vegetables 4.0%
Breads, pasta 11.0%
Meats, poultry, fish 10.0%
Shortening, oils 5.0%
Milk, butter, cheese 20.0%

6. Discuss the results.

Variations:
1. Invite a math teacher in to help plot the results, or do this as a combined lesson and team teach.

2. Use magazines and plot the percentage of space devoted to food ads.

3. Videotape commercials and play the tape so the entire class can work out the results together.

FOOD ADS Checklist (DN-61)

DIRECTIONS: Watch television for 1 hour and list the food ads on the chart in the proper categories. Time each commercial and bring your results to class.

Category	Product	Length of Ad
Sugars, Desserts, Snacks, Soft Drinks		
Milk, Butter, Cheese, Yogurt		
Meats, Poultry, Fish		
Breads, Pasta, Cereal		
Oils, Butters, Sauces, Mayonnaise		
Fruits, Vegetables		

FOOD ADS Pie Chart (DN-62)

DIRECTIONS: Write in the percentages of air time devoted to each category of food. Use your completed Food Ads Checklist (DN-61) for the information needed. Color code and label the graph.

☐ **Sugars, desserts, snacks, soft drinks**

☐ **Milk, butter, cheese, yogurt**

☐ **Meats, poultry, fish**

☐ **Breads, pasta, cereal**

☐ **Oils, butters, sauces, mayonnaise**

☐ **Fruits, vegetables**

Name _____ **Date** _____

TV SIGN-UP SHEET (DN-63)

TIME	MON	TUE	WED	THU	FRI	SAT	SUN
8:00–9:00 a.m.							
9:00–10:00 a.m.							
10:00–11:00 a.m.							
11:00–12 noon							
12:00–1:00 p.m.							
1:00–2:00 p.m.							
2:00–3:00 p.m.							
3:00–4:00 p.m.							
4:00–5:00 p.m.							
5:00–6:00 p.m.							
6:00–7:00 p.m.							
7:00–8:00 p.m.							
8:00–9:00 p.m.							
9:00–10:00 p.m.							
10:00–11:00 p.m.							

WEIGHT CONTROL

- **Caloric Intake and Expenditure**

- **Weight Guidelines**

- **Dieting**

CALORIES AND BMR (DN-64)

DIRECTIONS: Listed below is an explanation of basal metabolic rate (BMR) and how to estimate it for yourself. Figure your BMR and answer the questions.

Basal metabolic rate (BMR) is the rate at which you use energy when completely at rest. BMR varies according to age, sex, weight, and body size and shape. To get a rough estimate of your BMR in calories per day:

EXAMPLE (100-pound girl):

GIRLS:
1. Take your weight and add a zero: _____ 1000
2. Add your weight to that figure: + _____ +100
3. This is your approximate BMR: _____ 1,100 cal/day

EXAMPLE (150-pound boy)

BOYS:
1. Take your weight and add a zero: _____ 1500
2. Double your weight and add it: + _____ +300
3. This is your approximate BMR: _____ 1,800 cal/day

Calories are a measure of heat energy released when nutrients are burned or broken down. The more calories a food has, the more energy it contains. The number of calories a person needs in a day depends on many factors, such as amount of activity, air temperature, and BMR.

There are 3,500 calories in a pound of fat. To lose a pound, you would have to burn up 3,500 more calories than you consume. To gain a pound, you would have to eat 3,500 more calories than you burn.

©1993 by The Center for Applied Research in Education

1. How is it possible to have a high calorie/low nutrient diet?

2. Does an active person need more or fewer calories per day? Explain.

3. How might outside air temperature affect calorie burning?

ACTIVITY 16: BALANCING ACT

Concept/Description: To maintain weight, caloric intake must be equal to caloric output.

Objective: For students to determine if they balanced their caloric intake and expenditure for a given day.

Materials:
Eat 'Em Up (Caloric Intake Diary) (DN-65)
Work 'Em Off (Caloric Output Diary) (DN-66)
Nutrition Table of Common Foods (DN-67 to DN-71)
Energy Expenditure Chart (DN-74)
Pens or pencils

Directions:
1. Give each student a Caloric Intake Diary and a Caloric Output Diary and have them keep track of all that they eat and drink for one full day and all the activity they perform for the same day.

2. Bring the results back to class and compute the calories in and out using the Nutrition Table of Common Foods and the Energy Expenditure Chart.

3. Explain to students that this is not an exact measurement and more accurate information can be obtained by keeping a record over a longer period of time.

4. Ask students to determine whether the calorie intake and output were equal.

5. Explain the following:

   If intake is equal to output, then weight remains the same.

   If intake is greater than output, then weight is gained.

   If intake is less than output, then weight is lost.

6. Discuss.

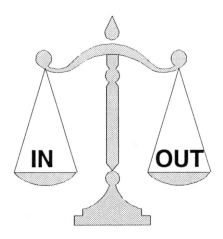

EAT 'EM UP (Caloric Intake Diary) (DN-65)

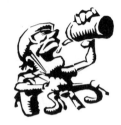

DIRECTIONS: Write down all the foods or drinks that you consume for one full day. Refer to the Nutrition Table of Common Foods (DN-67 to 71) and write down the approximate number of calories consumed for each food. Add up the total for the day.

Foods or Drinks	Amount	Calories Consumed

TOTAL_____

©1993 by The Center for Applied Research in Education

Name _____ **Date** _____

WORK 'EM OFF (Caloric Output Diary) (DN-66)

DIRECTIONS: Write down all the exercise that you do for one full day and the amount of time that you do it. Then, refer to the Energy Expenditure Chart (DN-74) and figure the approximate number of calories that you burned for each activity. Add up the total for the day.

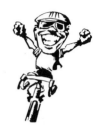

Activity	Amount of Time	Calories Burned

TOTAL_____

NUTRITION TABLE OF COMMON FOODS (DN-67)

Food	Amount	Calories
Almonds, whole	12 to 14	85
Apple	1 medium	70
Apple juice	½ cup	60
Applesauce:		
unsweetened	½ cup	50
sweetened	½ cup	115
Apricots:		
canned in syrup	½ cup	110
dried	5 halves	50
fresh	3 medium	50
Apricot nectar	½ cup	70
Asparagus	4 medium stalks	10
Avocado	½ 10-ounce avocado	185
Bacon:		
crisp, fried	2 slices	90
Canadian, uncooked	3 ounces	185
Banana	1 medium	100
Bagel	1 medium (2 ounces)	160
Beans, cooked:		
green, fresh or frozen	½ cup	15
limas, fresh or frozen	½ cup	95
wax, fresh, frozen	½ cup	45
Beans, kidney, canned	1 cup	230
Beef, broiled meat only:		
ground, lean	3 ounces	185
round, lean	3 ounces	160
sirloin, lean	3 ounces	185
Beets, fresh	2 (½ cup dried)	25
Biscuits:		
baking powder	1 (2-inch diameter)	90
refrigerator	1 biscuit	
Blueberries, fresh or frozen, unsweetened	½ cup	40
Bologna (all-meat)	1 ounce	80
Bouillon cubes	1 cube	5
Breads, one-ounce slice:		
French or Italian	1 slice	65
rye	1 slice	60
white	1 slice	70
white, raisin	1 slice	65
whole wheat	1 slice	65
Bread crumbs, dry	¼ cup	100
Broccoli, fresh or frozen, cooked	1 cup	20
Brussel sprouts, fresh or frozen, cooked	1 cup	55
Butter	1 tablespoon	100
Cabbage, fresh:		
boiled	½ cup	15
raw	½ cup (shredded)	10
Cakes:		
angel food	1/12 of 10-inch cake	135
chiffon	1/16 of 10-inch cake	215
chocolate cake, fudge frosting	1/16 of a 9-inch layer cake	235

©1993 by The Center for Applied Research in Education

Source: Abstracted from publications issued by U.S. Department of Agriculture and data submitted by food manufacturers.

Food	Amount	Calories
cupcake, plain	1 medium	90
yellow cake, fudge frosting	¹⁄₁₆ of a 9-inch layer cake	275
Candy:		
caramel, plain	1 piece	40
chocolate, milk	1 ounce	145
gum drop	1 small	10
sour ball	1 large	35
peanut brittle	1 ounce	120
Canteloupe	½ (5-inch diameter)	60
Carrots:		
cooked	½ cup sliced	20
raw	1 5½″ × 1″ carrot	20
Catsup	1 tablespoon	15
Cauliflower, cooked	½ cup	15
Celery, raw	1 large stalk	15
Cereals, ready-to-eat:		
All-Bran flakes	1 ounce	70
corn flakes	1 ounce	110
puffed rice, wheat	1 ounce	110
Rice Krispies	1 ounce	110
Raisin Bran	1 ounce	105
Shredded Wheat	1 ounce	110
Cheese:		
American, processed	1 ounce	105
cheddar	1 ounce	115
cheese spread	1 ounce	80
cottage, creamed	⅓ cup	85
cream	2 tablespoons (1 ounce)	105
mozzarella, whole milk	1 ounce	90
parmesan or romano, grated	2 tablespoons	50
ricotta, partially skimmed milk	⅓ cup	85
Roquefort or bleu	1 ounce	105
Swiss, processed or natural	1 ounce	105
Cherries:		
canned in syrup	½ cup	115
fresh, sweet	½ cup	40
Chicken, fryers, uncooked:		
breast, with skin	1 whole (¾ pound)	295
leg and thigh, with skin	1 small (½ pound)	190
light meat, without skin	4 ounces	115
dark meat, without skin	4 ounces	130
Chocolate:		
milk	1 ounce	145
semi-sweet	1 ounce	145
Chocolate pudding	½ cup	175
Cod, uncooked	4 ounces	90
Cola drinks	8 ounces	90
Collards, cooked	½ cup	25
Cookies:		
chocolate chip	1 (1-inch diameter)	50
fig bar	1 square	50
ginger snap	1 small (2-inch diameter)	30
oatmeal	1 large (3-inch diameter)	65
sandwich, creme	1 cookie	50
vanilla wafer	1 cookie	20

Food	Amount	Calories
Corn, cooked:		
canned, whole kernel	½ cup	85
fresh or frozen	1 ear (5-inches long)	70
Cornmeal, uncooked	1 cup	500
Crackers:		
graham	4 (2½-inch diameter)	110
oyster	10 crackers	45
rye wafer	2 wafers	45
saltine	4 squares	50
Cranberries, raw	1 cup	45
Cranberry sauce	2 tablespoons	40
Cream:		
half-and-half	1 tablespoon	20
heavy	1 tablespoon	55
	1 cup	840
light	1 tablespoon	30
	1 cup	505
sour	1 tablespoon	25
Cream of Wheat, dry	1 ounce	100
Cucumber, raw	1 medium (10 ounces)	43
Danish pastry, plain	4½-inch piece	275
Doughnut, cake-type	1 medium	125
Egg, raw	1 medium	70
Eggplant, cooked	1 cup, diced	40
Flounder, raw	4 ounces	90
Flour:		
all-purpose	1 cup	420
whole-wheat	1 cup	400
Frankfurter, all-meat	1.6-ounce frankfurter	135
Fruit cocktail, canned	½ cup	95
Gelatin dessert	½ cup	70
Gelatin, unflavored, dry	1 envelope	25
Grapefruit	½ medium	45
Grapefruit juice	½ cup	50
Grape juice	½ cup	85
Grapes	20 grapes	50
Gravy, canned beef	2 tablespoons	15
Haddock, uncooked	4 ounces	90
Halibut, uncooked	4 ounces	115
Ham, boiled	1 ounce	70
Honey	1 tablespoon	65
Ice cream, vanilla (10% butterfat)	1 cup	255
Ice milk, vanilla	1 cup	200
Jam or jelly	1 tablespoon	55
Lamb chop, lean, cooked	4 ounces (with bone)	140
Lemon or lime juice	¼ cup	15
Lentils, dried, raw	2½ tablespoons	85
Lettuce, raw	1 cup, chopped	10
Liver, uncooked:		
beef or calf	4 ounces	155
chicken	4 ounces	145
Lobster, cooked meat	3 ounces	80
Macaroni and cheese	1 cup	430
Macaroni, uncooked	1 ounce (½ cup cooked)	105
Margarine	1 tablespoon	100
Mars hmallows, plain	1 average	25

Food	Amount	Calories
Matzoh, plain	1 regular	120
Milk:		
buttermilk	1 cup	90
condensed, sweetened	½ cup	490
evaporated, undiluted	½ cup	175
low fat, 1% fat	1 cup	105
skimmed	1 cup	90
whole, 3.5% fat	1 cup	160
Milk, dry, non-fat instant	⅓ cup (makes 1 cup liquid)	80
Molasses, light	1 tablespoon	50
Muffins:		
corn	1 (2⅜-inch diameter)	125
bran	1 (3-inch diameter)	105
English	1 (3½-inch diameter)	140
Mushrooms:		
canned	1 cup (solids and liquid)	40
fresh	1 pound	125
Noodles, uncooked	1 ounce (½ cup cooked)	110
Oatmeal, uncooked	1 ounce (¾ cup cooked)	105
Oils, vegetable:		
corn, cottonseed, olive, soybean, etc.	1 tablespoon	125
Olives, green, pitted	4 medium	20
Onion, raw	1 medium	40
Orange	1 medium	65
Orange juice, fresh, frozen, canned	½ cup	55
Pancakes, from mix	2 (4-inch diameter)	120
Parsley, raw	5 tablespoons, chopped	5
Pea, green:		
canned	½ cup	60
frozen	½ cup	60
Pea, split dry	½ cup	345
Peach nectar	½ cup	60
Peaches:		
canned, syrup pack	½ cup halves with syrup	100
fresh	1 medium	35
Peanuts, roasted	8 to 10	55
Peanut butter	1 tablespoon	95
Pears:		
canned, syrup pack	½ cup halves with syrup	100
fresh	1 medium	100
Pecans	9 medium halves	70
Peppers, green	1 medium	15
Pickle, dill	1 (4″ × 1¾″ pickle)	15
Pie crust, made with vegetable shortening:		
homemade, single crust	1 9-inch shell	900
Pies:		
apple, double crust	⅙ of 9-inch pie	405
cherry, double crust	⅙ of 9-inch pie	410
custard	⅙ of 9-inch pie	330
lemon meringue	⅙ of 9-inch pie	355
pecan	⅙ of 9-inch pie	575
Pineapple, canned:		
slices, syrup-pack	2 slices	90
slices, juice-pack	2 slices	65
Pineapple juice	½ cup	65
Pizza, cheese	⅛ of 14-inch pie	185

NUTRITION TABLE OF COMMON FOODS (*continues*) (DN-71)

Food	Amount	Calories
Plums:		
canned syrup pack	½ cup with syrup	100
fresh	1 (2-inch diameter)	25
Popcorn, popped	1 cup	25
Pork, roasted meat only		
ham, cured, lean	3 ounces	210
ham, fresh, lean	3 ounces	185
loin chop, lean	3 ounces	230
Potatoes:		
baked	1 medium	90
boiled, pared	1 medium	90
french-fried	10 pieces	155
Soups:		
chicken-noodle	1 serving	55
Manhattan clam chowder	1 serving	65
minestrone	1 serving	85
mushroom, cream of	1 serving	185
tomato	1 serving	70
vegetable	1 serving	60
Spinach, frozen, cooked	½ cup	20
Squash, cooked:		
summer	½ cup	15
winter	½ cup	65
Strawberries, fresh	½ cup	25
Sugar:		
brown	1 cup	820
granulated	1 cup	770
	1 tablespoon	40
powdered	1 cup	460
Sunflower seeds, shelled	1 tablespoon	45
Syrup, maple	1 tablespoon	50
Tangerine	1 (2½-inch diameter)	40
Tomato juice	½ cup	25
Tomatoes:		
canned	½ cup	25
fresh	1 medium	40
Tuna, canned:		
oil-pack	6½-ounce can	530
water-pack	6½-ounce can	235
Turkey, roasted:		
light meat	4 ounces	200
dark meat	4 ounces	230
Veal, roasted	4 ounces	185
Vegetable juice	½ cup	20
Waffle	1 7-inch waffle	205
Walnuts, English	8 halves	50
Watermelon	1 wedge, 4″ × 8″	115
Wheat germ	1 tablespoon	15
Whipped topping, frozen	1 tablespoon	15
Yogurt, plain	1 cup	150

CALORIE TALLY (DN-72)

DIRECTIONS: Listed below are some fast foods with their amount of calories. Using a red crayon or colored pencil, fill in the graph for each food. The first one is done for you.

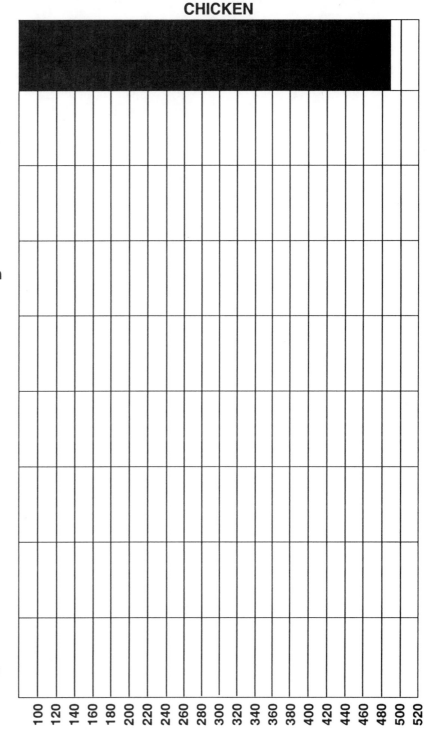

CHICKEN

Arby's Chicken Breast Sandwich (489)

Burger King BK Broiler Chicken Sandwich (379)

Dairy Queen Grilled Chicken (300)

Hardee's Grilled Chicken Breast Sandwich (310)

Kentucky Fried Chicken Skin-Free Breast (220)

Kentucky Fried Chicken Original Recipe Breast (260)

McDonald's McChicken Sandwich (415)

Taco Bell Chicken Burrito (334)

Wendy's Grilled Chicken Sandwich (340)

100 120 140 160 180 200 220 240 260 280 300 320 340 360 380 400 420 440 460 480 500 520

CALORIE TALLY, TOO (DN-73)

DIRECTIONS: With a partner, research the number of calories in some fast foods and write down similar products from different restaurants (McDonald's, Wendy's, Burger King, etc.). Color in the graph showing the number of calories in each and compare. What would cause similar products to differ in the amount of calories? Refer to Calorie Tally (DN-72) for an example of a calorie graph.

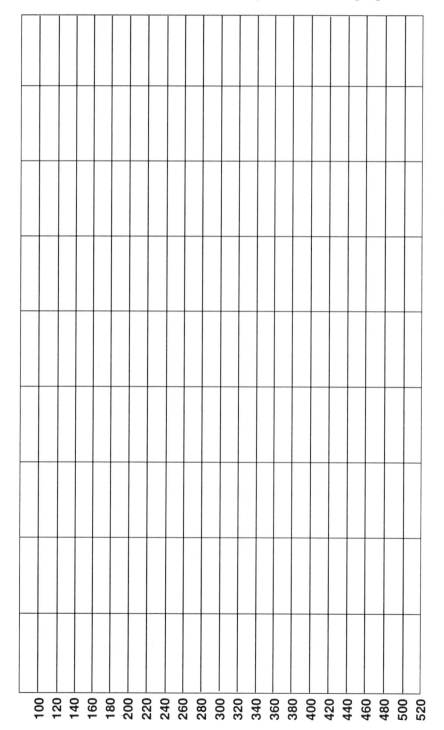

100 120 140 160 180 200 220 240 260 280 300 320 340 360 380 400 420 440 460 480 500 520

ENERGY EXPENDITURE BY A 150-POUND PERSON IN VARIOUS ACTIVITIES (DN-74)

Activity	Gross Energy Spent in Calories Per Hour
Rest and light activity	**50–200**
Lying down or sleeping	80
Sitting	100
Driving an automobile	120
Standing	140
Domestic work	180
Moderate activity	**200–350**
Bicycling (5½ mph)	210
Walking (2½ mph)	210
Gardening	220
Canoeing (2½ mph)	230
Golf	250
Lawn mowing (power mower)	250
Bowling	270
Lawn mowing (hand mower)	270
Fencing	300
Rowboating (2½ mph)	300
Swimming (¼ mph)	300
Walking (3¼ mph)	300
Badminton	350
Horseback riding (trotting)	350
Square dancing	350
Volleyball	350
Roller skating	350
Vigorous activity	**over 350**
Table tennis	360
Ditch digging (hand shovel)	400
Ice skating (10 mph)	400
Wood chopping or sawing	400
Tennis	420
Water skiing	480
Hill climbing (100 ft. per hr.)	490
Skiing (10 mph)	600
Squash and handball	600
Cycling (13 mph)	660
Scull rowing (race)	840
Running (10 mph)	900

Source: President's Council on Physical Fitness and Sports, "Exercise and Weight Control," (Washington, D.C.: U.S. Government Printing Office, 1979).

HEIGHT-WEIGHT CHART (DN-75)

Many people have written diet books and diet plans. Magazines constantly advertise "miracle" weight-loss plans, yet people are still struggling with weight. The only sure way to lose weight is to use up more calories than you consume.

To help you determine your ideal weight, refer to the chart below. Remember to always check with your physician before starting any weight-loss program.

HEIGHT AND WEIGHT TABLES*

Weights at ages 25-59 based on lowest mortality. Weight in pounds according to frame (in indoor clothing weighing 5 lbs. for men and 3 lbs. for women; shoes with 1″ heels).

MEN Height Feet Inches	Small Frame	Medium Frame	Large Frame	WOMEN Height Feet Inches	Small Frame	Medium Frame	Large Frame
5 2	128-134	131-141	138-150	4 10	102-111	109-121	118-131
5 3	130-136	133-143	140-153	4 11	103-113	111-123	120-134
5 4	132-138	135-145	142-156	5 0	104-115	113-126	122-137
5 5	134-140	137-148	144-160	5 1	106-118	115-129	125-140
5 6	136-142	139-151	146-164	5 2	108-121	118-132	128-143
5 7	138-145	142-154	149-168	5 3	111-124	121-135	131-147
5 8	140-148	145-157	152-172	5 4	114-127	124-138	134-151
5 9	142-151	148-160	155-176	5 5	117-130	127-141	137-155
5 10	144-154	151-163	158-180	5 6	120-133	130-144	140-159
5 11	146-157	154-166	161-184	5 7	123-136	133-147	143-163
6 0	149-160	157-170	164-188	5 8	126-139	136-150	146-167
6 1	152-164	160-174	168-192	5 9	129-142	139-153	149-170
6 2	155-168	164-178	172-197	5 10	132-145	142-156	152-173
6 3	158-172	167-182	176-202	5 11	135-148	145-159	155-176
6 4	162-176	171-187	181-207	6 0	138-151	148-162	158-179

©1993 by The Center for Applied Research in Education

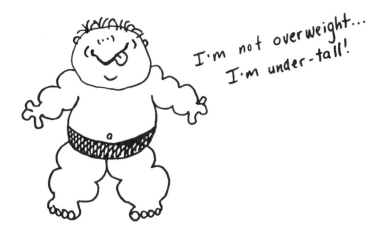

*Used with permission of Metropolitan Life Insurance Company

Name _____ **Date** _____

FITNESS OR FATNESS? QUIZ (DN-76)

DIRECTIONS: How much do you know about fitness? Take the quiz below by placing a *T* for true or an *F* for false in the blank.

_____ 1. To get the most benefits from exercising, it is necessary to exercise at least one hour every day.

_____ 2. To increase the size of your leg muscles, you should lift weights every day to exercise the same group of muscles.

_____ 3. If you stop exercising, your present level of fitness will begin to drop after only one week of inactivity.

_____ 4. For static stretches to increase flexibility, they must be held for 15 to 20 seconds.

_____ 5. Women who lift weights will develop huge muscles and look masculine.

_____ 6. It is best to eat sugar or sweets before competition to give yourself plenty of energy for a long period of time.

_____ 7. Take salt tablets when you exercise in hot weather.

_____ 8. Don't drink water when working out; it can cause cramps.

_____ 9. It is better to eat a banana to replace potassium than to drink a sports drink before competition.

_____10. Target heart rate is 60% to 75% of your maximum heart rate and is the heart rate you should attain and stay at during an aerobic workout.

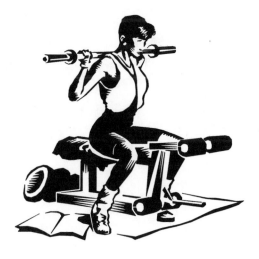

HAZARDS OF OBESITY (DN-77)

Obesity occurs when there is an excess of fat, or adipose tissue, in the body. Adipose tissue is a type of connective tissue in which many cells are filled with fat. The body needs adipose tissue, but too much can result in serious health problems. Some of the dangers are listed below:

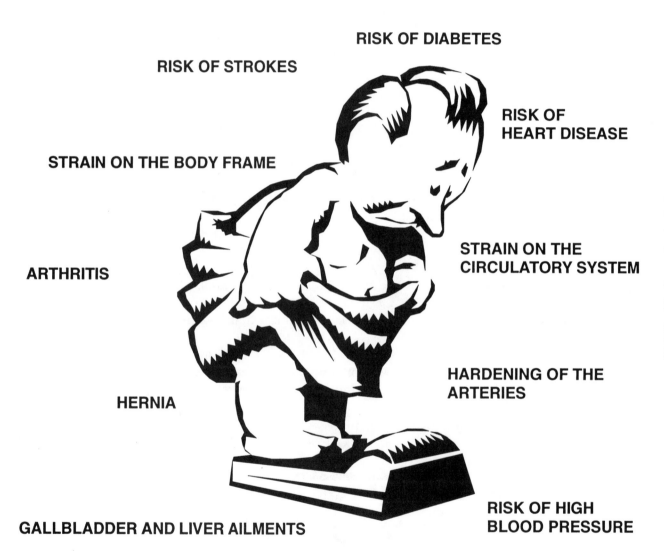

RISK OF DIABETES

RISK OF STROKES

RISK OF HEART DISEASE

STRAIN ON THE BODY FRAME

STRAIN ON THE CIRCULATORY SYSTEM

ARTHRITIS

HARDENING OF THE ARTERIES

HERNIA

RISK OF HIGH BLOOD PRESSURE

GALLBLADDER AND LIVER AILMENTS

RISK OF APPENDICITIS

WEIGHT CONTROL HINTS (DN-78)

DIRECTIONS: Listed below are some suggestions for controlling your weight safely. Add your own to the bottom of the list.

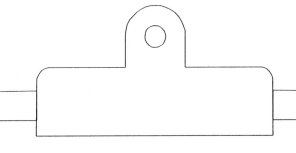

1. Drink a large glass of water before meals. It helps fill the stomach and you won't feel like overeating.
2. Use a smaller plate to make the portions look larger.
3. Don't skip meals. Eat six small meals instead of three large ones. Don't eat more food, just divide it into six meals.
4. Keep a chart of your weight progress, but don't weigh yourself more than once a week.
5. Eat slowly and chew food thoroughly. It takes 20 minutes for your stomach to signal your brain that you are feeling full.
6. Put a motivational picture or sign on your refrigerator.
7. Trade high-calorie foods for lower-calorie foods. Eat popcorn instead of potato chips or a baked potato instead of fries.

Your Suggestions:

8.

9.

10.

11.

12.

TRUE–FALSE DIETING QUIZ (DN-79)

DIRECTIONS: How much do you know about safe dieting? Place a *T* for true or an *F* for false in the blank to the left.

_____ 1. The body's need for food is far greater than its need for water.

_____ 2. Use the U.S. RDA to find the exact percentages of key nutrients you need.

_____ 3. Health experts recommend that you not lose more than 1½ pounds to 2 pounds per week when on a diet.

_____ 4. People who are extremely underweight can have as many problems as people who are overweight.

_____ 5. If you eat more calories than you burn, you will lose weight.

_____ 6. There are 1000 calories in one pound of fat.

_____ 7. Even a small amount of exercise can help speed up your metabolic rate.

_____ 8. When you diet, the first weight to be lost will be fat.

_____ 9. The pinch test and skin caliper test are used to measure the amount of muscle under the skin.

_____ 10. Diuretics are medications that cause the body to lose water weight.

ACTIVITY 17: DIET SPY

**Concept/
Description:** The purpose of a successful diet is to take weight off safely and to keep the weight off. Many commercial diet plans are inadequate and sometimes dangerous.

Objective: To analyze specific diet plans and determine their safeness and effectiveness.

Materials: Diet Plan Analysis Sheet (DN-80)
Various diet plan literature or videos
Pens or pencils

Directions:
1. Have students bring in diet plan literature or videos.
2. Give each group of three to four a Diet Plan Analysis Sheet.
3. Have students analyze a diet plan and answer the questions on the sheet.
4. Have a spokesperson from each group briefly explain the idea behind the plan and tell whether the group thinks the plan is safe and effective and why or why not.
5. Discuss that the only safe and effective way to lose weight is to:
   a. eat less
   b. eat a balanced diet
   c. exercise
   d. change eating habits

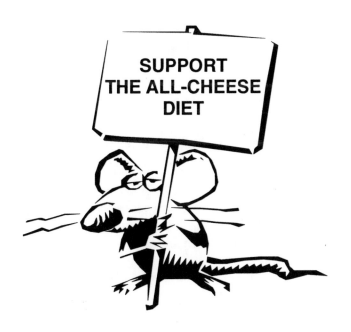

SUPPORT
THE ALL-CHEESE
DIET

DIET PLAN ANALYSIS SHEET (DN-80)

1. What is the background of the author or inventor of the diet? What makes that person an "expert" in the field of nutrition?

2. What is the main idea of the diet?

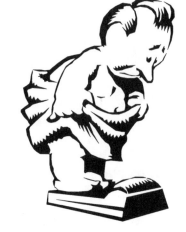

3. Does the diet promote or encourage exercise? Explain.

4. Does the diet give tips on how to change eating habits? If so, give an example.

5. Does the diet use a variety of foods from all food groups?

6. Does the diet list any precautions or warnings? If so, what are they?

7. Does the diet encourage eating at least 1,200 calories per day?

8. Does your group recommend this diet? Why or why not? Explain.

EATING DISORDERS

- Anorexia and Bulimia

- Media's Role

EATING DISORDERS: Anorexia Nervosa (DN-81)

DIRECTIONS: Research the eating disorder Anorexia Nervosa and answer the questions.

1. What is ANOREXIA NERVOSA?

2. What are some of the possible causes?

3. What are the signs and symptoms?

4. What are the health risks?

5. Where, in your community, can you get help for eating disorders?

EATING DISORDERS: Bulimia (DN-82)

DIRECTIONS: Research the eating disorder BULIMIA and answer the questions.

1. What is BULIMIA?

2. What are some of the possible causes?

3. What are the signs and symptoms?

4. What are the health risks?

5. Where, in your community, can you get help for eating disorders?

ACTIVITY 18: HEY GOOD LOOKIN', WHAT'S COOKIN'?

Concept/Description: Society has conditioned people, especially females, to believe that thin is beautiful.

Objective: To recognize the effect the media has had on body image and self-concept.

Materials: Hey, Baby... (DN-83)
Magazine ads of attractive models advertising any product
Pens or pencils

Directions:
1. Divide the class into pairs and give each pair a magazine ad showing an attractive model.
2. Ask pairs to look at the ad and fill in the Hey, Baby... worksheet.
3. When all have finished analyzing their ads, have pairs show their ads and briefly describe their findings.
4. Ask students if they feel these images are realistic and whether this could contribute to eating disorders. Discuss.
5. Although most anorexics and bulimics are girls, some are boys. Ask the class why they feel there are more girls than boys suffering from eating disorders. Discuss.

Variations:
1. Videotape TV commercials of "beautiful people" and analyze them as a class.
2. Have students make up their own commercials emphasizing the use of "beautiful people" to advertise anything from automobiles to food.
3. Have students videotape public address announcements highlighting the dangers of eating disorders. Play them for the class.

**DRINK
HIGH-SOCIETY
COLA**

**It's what the beautiful
people drink!**

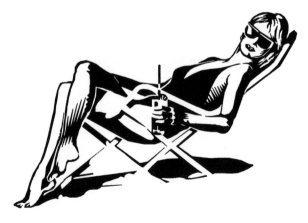

114

Name _____ **Date** _____

HEY, BABY... (DN-83)

DIRECTIONS: Analyze the advertisement given to you and answer the questions.

1. Describe the people shown in your advertisement.

No one asks me to do their ads.....

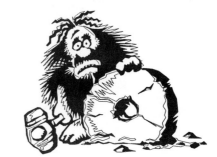

2. What product is being advertised?

3. Is the emphasis in your ad on the product or the people?

4. Why do you think the advertiser used those particular people in the ad? What does the ad seem to imply?

5. Do you think the people in the ad represent typical Americans? Why or why not?

6. Do you think people tend to compare themselves to the images the media portrays?

7. How can associating beautiful people with products help to sell the products?

8. Do you think the media has contributed to some people having eating disorders? Why or why not? Explain.

GENERAL
ACTIVITIES

ACTIVITY 19: FULL OF BALONEY!

Concept/
Description: Over the years, food has become a common way to describe a person or a person's qualities or behavior, or a situation.

Objective: To be the group that comes up with the most food-related expressions.

Materials: Paper
Pens or pencils

Directions:
1. Divide the class into groups of three to four.
2. On the signal, have students write down as many food-related expressions as they can think of. Examples are provided on the Food Expressions Sheet (DN-84).
3. The group that comes up with the most is the winner.

    Note: Be sure to insist that all terms be acceptable for a classroom setting. Any inappropriate comments will be "squashed."

    (Sorry, I couldn't help myself!)
4. Ask students why they think it is common to use food to express feelings.
5. Discuss.

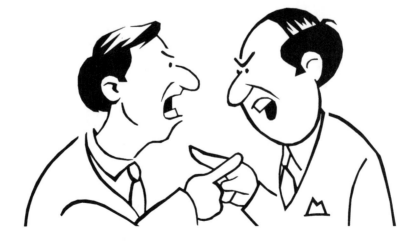

GET OFF MY CASE, POTATO FACE!

KNOCK IT OFF, MEATHEAD!

FOOD EXPRESSIONS SHEET (DN-84)

Here are some expressions related to food:

cool as a cucumber

acts like a hot dog

you bought a lemon

in a jam

in a pickle

top banana

plum job

full of beans

full of bologna

full of soup

you're chicken

in a stew

it's a piece of cake

earn the bread

earn the dough

bring home the bacon

smart cookie

egghead

sour grapes

cream of the crop

corny joke

good egg

that's peachy

ham it up

cauliflower ear

she's a little shrimp

flat as a pancake

something's fishy

easy as pie

cut the mustard

I'm on a roll

bust your chops

crabby

I don't relish the idea

apple of my eye

butter up the teacher

two peas in a pod

bowl of cherries

What am I, chopped liver?

all clammed-up

face is beet red

not my cup of tea

doesn't mince any words

sit and vegetate

nutty

nutty as a fruitcake

turkey

cold turkey

peaches-and-cream complexion

give him the raspberries

couch potato

pudding of a job

spicy novel

a real honey

he was sauced

squash that idea

that's the way the cookie crumbles

slow as molasses

NUTRITION CROSSWORD PUZZLE (DN-85)

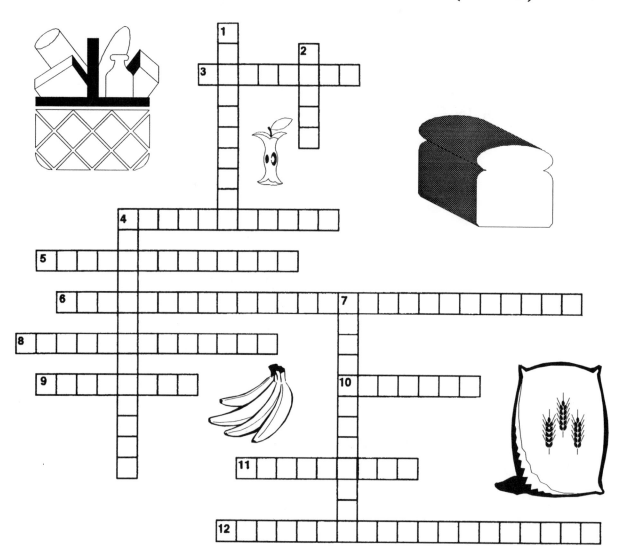

DOWN

1. Building blocks of protein
2. The nondigestible part of certain foods that aids in moving food through the digestive tract
4. Chemical compounds that are converted to glycogen when broken down during digestion
7. Special molecules that carry cholesterol through the bloodstream

ACROSS

3. Organic compounds that work with enzymes to promote chemical changes
4. Fatty substance found in all animal tissue
5. Fatty acid with as many hydrogen atoms as it can hold
6. A general guide to the amount of nutrients needed daily
8. Three fatty acids attached to one glycerol molecule
9. Inorganic substances formed in the earth with distinct chemical and physical properties
10. The second most abundant substance in the human body and a vital part of every cell
11. Chemical substances obtained from food during digestion
12. Fatty acid that has room for four or more hydrogen atoms

NUTRITION MATCH-UP (DN-86)

DIRECTIONS: Match the correct term with its definition by placing the correct letter in the blank to the left. Not all terms will be used.

_____ 1. Losing and gaining weight repeatedly

_____ 2. A unit of energy

_____ 3. Serious illness from overeating and self-induced vomiting

_____ 4. Abnormal loss of body fluids

_____ 5. Eating plan that requires cutting down on salt

_____ 6. Eating plan limiting foods high in animal and other saturated fats

_____ 7. Last date a product should be used

_____ 8. Bacteria found in improperly canned foods that can cause illness and death

_____ 9. Foods relatively low in fat

_____ 10. Food that uses the entire kernel and contains most of the original nutrients

a. botulism
b. dehydration
c. chicken, turkey (skinless)
d. beef, pork
e. nutrition label
f. unit pricing
g. expiration date
h. low-sodium diet
i. low-cholesterol diet
j. setpoint
k. yo-yo dieting
l. crash dieting
m. anorexia
n. bulimia
o. perfringen poisoning
p. whole wheat bread
q. white bread
r. calorie

CROSSED UP! (DN-87)

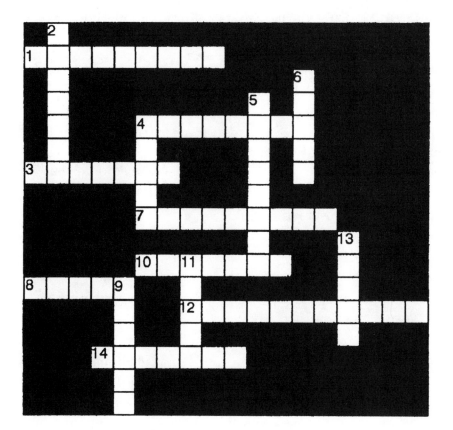

ACROSS

1. Substances added to food
3. Exercise that increases oxygen intake to stimulate the heart and lungs
4. Blood vessels that carry blood from the heart to the body
7. Process by which cells use oxygen to turn food into energy
8. Mixture of gastric juices and food in the stomach
10. Blood sugar
12. Substance found in blood, tissues, and digestive juices, too much of which can cause heart disease
14. A muscle that separates the stomach from the small intestine

DOWN

2. Body cells that store fat
4. Protein building blocks: _____ acids
5. Illness where the pancreas does not make enough insulin
6. The rate at which the body uses energy for its basic processes: _____ metabolic rate (BMR)
9. Substance that speeds up a chemical process
11. Stomach sore
13. Carbohydrate found in plant foods that helps the digestive system work more smoothly

ANSWER KEYS TO REPRODUCIBLES

BREAKDOWN (DN-1)

DIRECTIONS: The purpose of the digestive system is to break down food into simple molecules that pass into the bloodstream to provide the body with energy for life. Label the parts of the digestive system on the diagram below. Use the words in the box to help you.

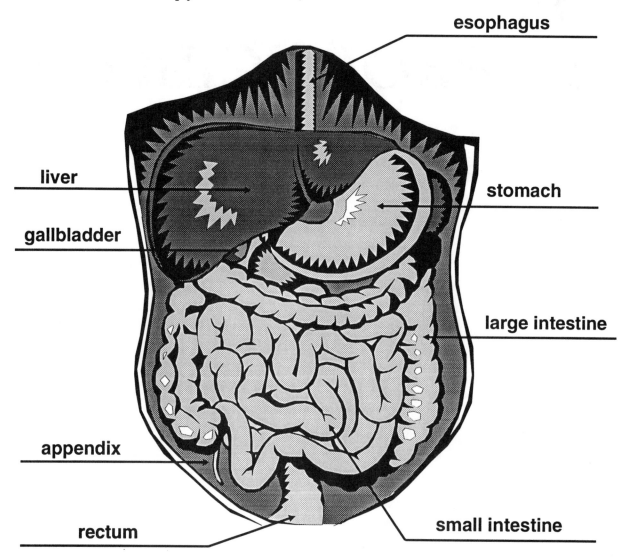

esophagus

liver

gallbladder

stomach

large intestine

appendix

rectum

small intestine

appendix	large intestine
gallbladder	rectum
liver	esophagus
stomach	small intestine

AS THE STOMACH CHURNS (DN-2)

DIRECTIONS: Label the parts of the digestive system shown below. Use the words in the box.

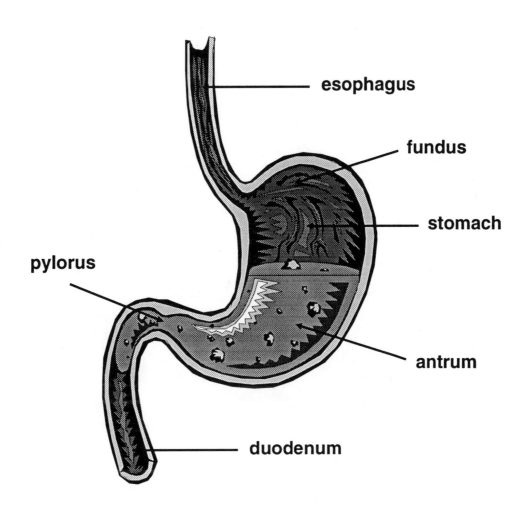

esophagus
fundus
stomach
pylorus
antrum
duodenum

esophagus
fundus
duodenum
pylorus
stomach
antrum

LIVER, GALLBLADDER, AND PANCREAS (DN-3)

DIRECTIONS: The liver, gallbladder, and pancreas are aids in the digestive process. Read about their functions in the boxes, then label the parts using the words in the box at the bottom of the sheet.

Gallbladder:
The gallbladder is a small sac that stores bile. The gallbladder is located on the underside of the liver.

Pancreas:
The pancreas produces alkaline enzymes that flow into the small intestine. The pancreas also produces insulin and glucagon.

Liver:
The liver, the largest gland in the body, has over 500 functions. Its major functions are:
1. Production of bile, a yellowish-green fluid that helps to break down fats.
2. Conversion of glucose to glycogen.
3. Balance of blood sugar in the body.
4. Helping to metabolize carbohydrates, fats, and proteins.
5. Changing toxic wastes into less toxic substances.
6. Stores fat-soluble vitamins A, D, E, and K and several water-soluble vitamins.

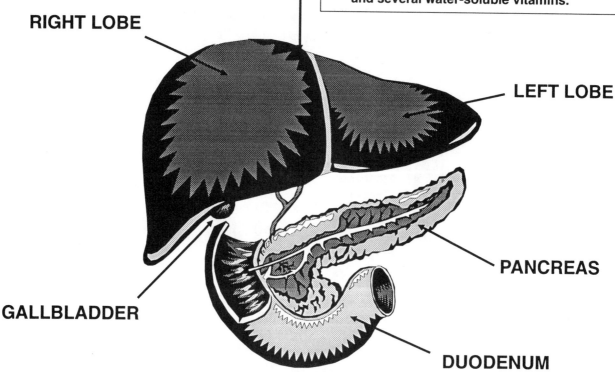

LIVER

RIGHT LOBE

LEFT LOBE

PANCREAS

GALLBLADDER

DUODENUM

liver	left lobe
gallbladder	right lobe
pancreas	duodenum

MUSCLE HUSTLE (DN-4)

DIRECTIONS: Label the parts of the muscular system below, by using the words in the box.

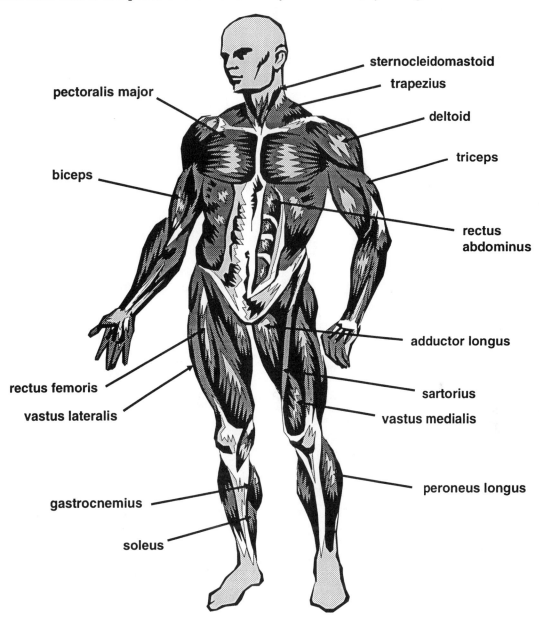

sternocleidomastoid

trapezius

pectoralis major

deltoid

triceps

biceps

rectus abdominus

adductor longus

rectus femoris

sartorius

vastus lateralis

vastus medialis

peroneus longus

gastrocnemius

soleus

pectoralis major	**sternocleidomastoid**	**rectus femoris**
peroneus longus	**trapezius**	**vastus lateralis**
vastus medialis	**deltoid**	**gastrocnemius**
sartorius	**biceps**	**rectus abdominus**
soleus	**triceps**	**adductor longus**

MUSCLE MADNESS (DN-5)

DIRECTIONS: Unscramble the underlined words to complete these sentences about the muscular system. Write your answer in the blank to the left of each sentence.

voluntary   1. Muscles that we can consciously move are called <u>RNOVLTUAY</u> muscles.

contraction   2. Shortening of the muscle that causes movement is called muscular <u>RACCONTTNIO</u>.

smooth   3. The muscles found in the walls of the stomach and intestines are called <u>MOOTHS</u> muscles.

skeletal   4. <u>LEKSELTA</u> muscles are responsible for movement of the body and limbs.

triceps   5. The muscle that straightens the arm is called the <u>SCITREP</u>.

fatigue   6. If the blood supply doesn't keep up with muscle activity, <u>UGTAFIE</u> is the result.

tendons   7. Muscles are connected to bones by <u>NENTOSD</u>.

biceps   8. The muscle that bends the arm at the elbow is the <u>SPCIBE</u>.

insertion   9. Skeletal muscles are attached to bones at two ends. One end is called the origin and the opposite end is the <u>NIESINTRO</u>.

tone   10. The ability of a muscle to stay tense is known as muscle <u>NOTE</u>.

©1993 by The Center for Applied Research in Education

CARBO CHARGED (DN-12)

Carbohydrates are starches and sugars that come mainly from plant food. Carbohydrates provide the body with much of the energy it needs each day. There are two types of carbohydrates: COMPLEX, or starches, and SIMPLE, or sugars.

DIRECTIONS: Fill in the words below to give some examples of some complex and simple carbohydrates.

Complex Carbohydrates:

1.   **M A** S **H E D**
2.   **Z I** T **I**
3.   **B** A **K E D**
4.   **B** R **E A D**
5.   C **R U S T**
6. **S P A G** H **E T T I**
7.   **W H** E **A T**
8. **R O L L** S

CLUES

1. Type of cooked potato
2. Type of pasta
3. Type of cooked potato
4. White, wheat, rye, etc.
5. Found on pizza, bread, rolls, etc.
6. Type of pasta
7. Type of whole-grain bread
8. Hard, dinner, crescent, etc.

CLUES

1. 7-Up, Coca-Cola, Mountain Dew, etc.
2. Refined, sweet substance found in the home
3. Kind of jelly
4. Kind of syrup
5. Fruit sugar
6. Milk sugar

Simple Carbohydrates:

1.   S **O F T** D **R I N K S**
2. **T A B L E** S U **G A R**
3.   G R **A P E**
4.   **M** A **P L E**
5.   **F** R **U C T O S E**
6.   **L A C** T **O S** E

Name _____ **Date** _____

FATTY BOOM-BA-LATTY (DN-13)

DIRECTIONS: For each item below, place an *X* in the box indicating which food you think contains more fat.

☐ 2 slices cheese pizza ☒ 1 fish sandwich	☒ 1 peanut butter and jelly sandwich ☐ 1 roasted pork chop
☐ 1 cup spaghetti and meatballs ☒ 1 small taco	☒ 10 french fries ☐ 10 baked potatoes
☒ 3 oz. fish sticks ☐ 2 sausage links	☒ 1/2 croissant ☐ 2 English muffins
☒ 1 regular cheeseburger ☐ 3 oz. sirloin steak	☒ 1/2 cup canned pudding ☐ 10-oz. vanilla milkshake
☐ 6 pancakes ☒ 1 cinnamon sweet roll	☒ 1 cup macaroni and cheese ☐ 10 slices bread
☐ 2 cups lowfat yogurt ☒ 1 tablespoon mayonnaise	☒ 1 oz. tortilla chips ☐ 1 cup unbuttered popcorn

FAT FACTS (DN-14)

DIRECTIONS: Find the letter that matches the number and fill it in on the blank line. Read the information about fat in the diet and discuss.

A	B	C	D	E	F	G	H	I	J	K	L	M
1	2	3	4	5	6	7	8	9	10	11	12	13

N	O	P	Q	R	S	T	U	V	W	X	Y	Z
14	15	16	17	18	19	20	21	22	23	24	25	26

The building blocks of fats are __F__ __A__ __T__ __T__ __Y__ acids. There are three types:
  6   1   20   20   25

monounsaturated, polyunsaturated, and __S__ __A__ __T__ __U__ __R__ __A__ __T__ __E__ __D__ . Fats that remain
  19   1   20   21   18   1   20   5   4

__L__ __I__ __Q__ __U__ __I__ __D__ at room temperature are either monounsaturated or polyunsaturated.
12   9   17   21   9   4

Some examples of polyunsaturated fats include oils made from __C__ __O__ __R__ __N__ safflower,
  3   15   18   14

sunflower, __S__ __O__ __Y__ __B__ __E__ __A__ __N__ cottonseed, and __S__ __E__ __S__ __A__ __M__ __E__ . Monounsaturated
  19   15   25   2   5   1   14   19   5   19   1   13   5

oils are __O__ __L__ __I__ __V__ __E__ , canola, avocado, and __P__ __E__ __A__ __N__ __U__ __T__ .
  15   12   9   22   5   16   5   1   14   21   20

More harmful because they cause the __L__ __I__ __V__ __E__ __R__ to produce too much
  12   9   22   5   18

__C__ __H__ __O__ __L__ __E__ __S__ __T__ __E__ __R__ __O__ __L__ are saturated fats, which remain __S__ __O__ __L__ __I__ __D__
  3   8   15   12   5   19   20   5   18   15   12   19   15   12   9   4

or semisolid at room temperature. Shortening and margarine are examples and are also referred

to as hydrogenated or partially hydrogenated. Many __A__ __N__ __I__ __M__ __A__ __L__ products are high in
  1   14   9   13   1   12

saturated fats, such as __B__ __E__ __E__ __F__ , pork, lamb, butter, __W__ __H__ __O__ __L__ __E__ milk, and dairy
  2   5   5   6   23   8   15   12   5

products from whole milk. Palm, palm-kernel, and __C__ __O__ __C__ __O__ __N__ __U__ __T__ oil are also high
  3   15   3   15   14   21   20

in saturated fats.

It's best to __C__ __U__ __T__ down on __A__ __L__ __L__ the fats and oils we eat to lower our risk of
  3   21   20   1   12   12

__H__ __E__ __A__ __R__ __T__ disease.
8   5   1   18   20

VITAMIN MATCH-UP (DN-17)

DIRECTIONS: Match the vitamin with its function by placing the name of the vitamin in the blank to the left. The vitamins are listed in the box.

B₁ (thiamine)	B₂ (riboflavin)	B₃ (niacin)	B₆ (pyridoxine)
B₁₂ (cobalamin)	folic acid	Biotin	pantothenic acid
C (ascorbic acid)	A	D	E K

A _____ 1. Maintains healthy skin, bones, and eyes.

K _____ 2. Aids in blood clotting.

pantothenic acid _____ 3. Aids in the functioning of the digestive tract.

B₁₂ _____ 4. Aids in red blood cell formation and synthesis of RNA and DNA.

B₃ _____ 5. Aids in digestion and carbohydrate use and is necessary for functioning of the nervous system.

Biotin _____ 6. Aids in metabolizing carbohydrates and other B vitamins.

C _____ 7. Aids in connective tissue, bone, tooth, and skin formation; resistance to infection; and iron assimilation.

B₆ _____ 8. Aids in protein, fat, and carbohydrate metabolism.

B₂ _____ 9. Aids in energy production in cells; promotes healthy skin.

folic acid _____ 10. Aids in blood cell formation, protein production, and enzyme functioning.

B₁ _____ 11. Aids in carbohydrate use; necessary for heart, nervous system, and appetite.

D _____ 12. Aids in calcium and phosphorous use.

E _____ 13. Aids in maintenance of vitamin A and fats.

PLUS AND MINUS (DN-18)

DIRECTIONS: Research the vitamins listed and write the problems that occur when there is a deficiency and an excess of each. Write your answers in the boxes. Note: In some cases, an excess of the vitamin does not cause problems, nor does it have any benefits. The body will rid itself of the excess.

VITAMIN	DEFICIENCY (−)	EXCESS (+)
A	Problems with night vision, infections of the mucous membranes, bone growth problems	Problems with vision, appetite, skin, joints, bones; nervous system damage
D	Rickets	Calcium deposits leading to deafness, kidney stones, and high blood pressure
K	Hemorrhage	**UNKNOWN**
Folic Acid	Anemia	— — —
B₆	Skin disorders	— — —
B₁₂	Anemia	— — —
C	Scurvy	Kidney stones, urinary tract infections
Niacin	Pellagra	Ulcers
Riboflavin	Skin disorders	— — —
Thiamine	Beriberi	— — —

DISSOLVE IN WATER (DN-19)

There are two classes of vitamins: fat-soluble and water-soluble. Fat-soluble vitamins are stored by the body and can be harmful if consumed in excess. Water-soluble vitamins are not stored by the body, so it is important that you eat foods that supply these vitamins every day.

DIRECTIONS: Write the fat-soluble vitamins in the fat molecule and the water-soluble vitamins in the water drop. Then, list some foods that supply you with each vitamin.

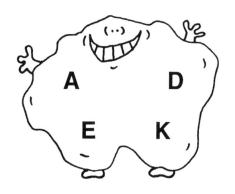
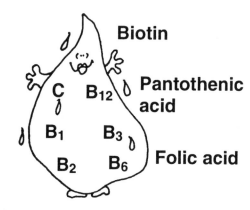

Vitamin A __liver, carrots, apricots, broccoli, milk__

Vitamin B_1 __pork, liver, oysters, legumes, wheat germ__

Vitamin K __green leafy vegetables, cauliflower, potatoes__

Vitamin B_{12} __meats, fish, poultry, dairy products__

Vitamin B_6 __meats, fish, poultry, oatmeal, potatoes__

Biotin __egg yolk, liver, mushrooms, peanuts__

Vitamin C __citrus fruits, broccoli, strawberries__

Vitamin D __sunlight, fortified milk, cod liver oil__

Vitamin E __vegetable oils, whole-grain bread, liver__

Pantothenic Acid __liver, kidneys, eggs, nuts, dark green vegetables__

Folic Acid __liver, wheat germ, eggs, kidneys__

Vitamin B_2 __milk, cheese, eggs, dried beans and peas__

Vitamin B_3 __liver, fish, poultry, eggs, peanuts__

ANATOMY OF A LUNCH (DN-23)

DIRECTIONS: Look at the lunch below. Next to each item, place the name of the food group to which each food belongs.

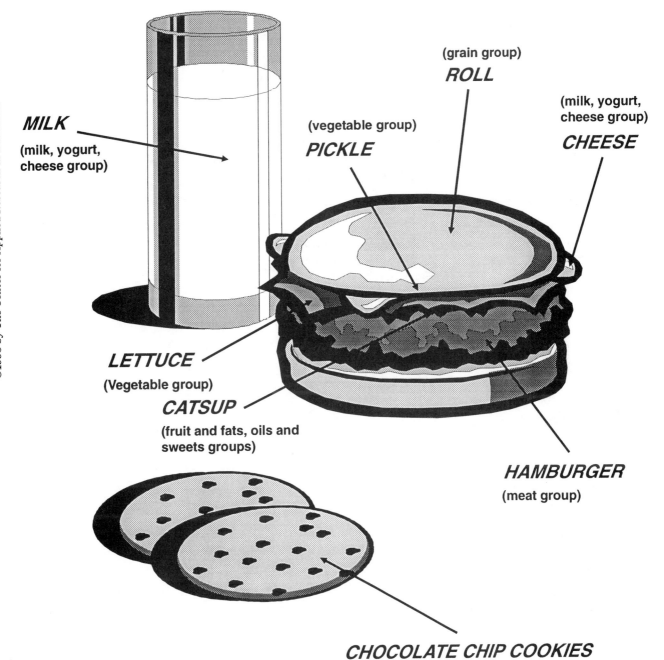

©1993 by The Center for Applied Research in Education

MILK
(milk, yogurt, cheese group)

(vegetable group)
PICKLE

(grain group)
ROLL

(milk, yogurt, cheese group)
CHEESE

LETTUCE
(Vegetable group)

CATSUP
(fruit and fats, oils and sweets groups)

HAMBURGER
(meat group)

CHOCOLATE CHIP COOKIES
(fats, oils, sweets group)

FOOD GUIDE PYRAMID (DN-32)

DIRECTIONS: Place each food in its proper area on the food pyramid by drawing a line from the food to the correct area. The Agriculture Department unveiled the pyramid as the new shape for the ideal American diet in place of the old pie chart.

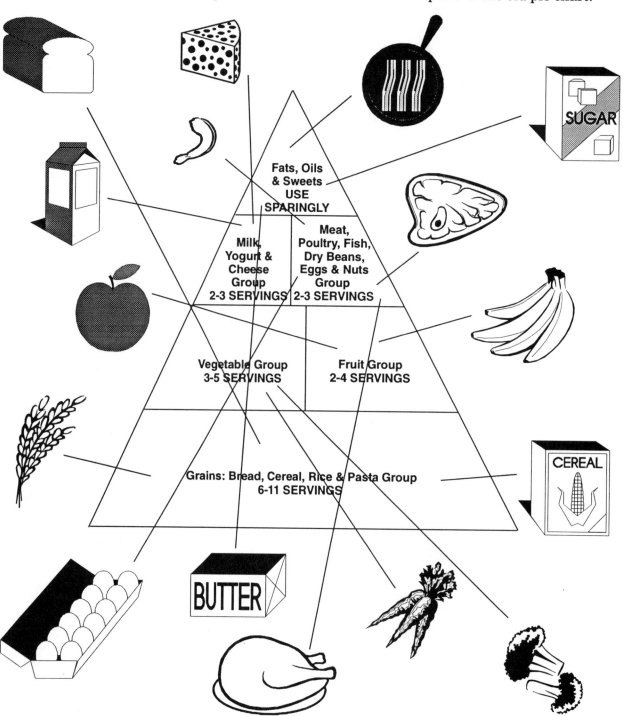

Fats, Oils & Sweets
USE SPARINGLY

Milk, Yogurt & Cheese Group
2-3 SERVINGS

Meat, Poultry, Fish, Dry Beans, Eggs & Nuts Group
2-3 SERVINGS

Vegetable Group
3-5 SERVINGS

Fruit Group
2-4 SERVINGS

Grains: Bread, Cereal, Rice & Pasta Group
6-11 SERVINGS

SUGAR

CEREAL

BUTTER

©1993 by The Center for Applied Research in Education

U.S. RDA INFORMATION SHEET (DN-33)

Many nutrients on a food label are listed as a percentage of the U.S. Recommended Daily Allowances. The U.S. RDA are the amount of nutrients needed each day by most healthy people.

The following are U.S. RDA for these nutrients:

PROTEIN	45 g
VITAMIN A	5000 IU
VITAMIN C	60 mg
THIAMIN	1.5 mg
RIBOFLAVIN	1.7 mg
NIACIN	20 mg
CALCIUM	1000 mg
IRON	18 mg

DIRECTIONS: Look at the food label below and answer the questions.

TONS-O-BRAN CEREAL

PERCENTAGES OF U.S.
RECOMMENDED DAILY ALLOWANCES

Protein	5 %
Vitamin A	25 %
Vitamin C	4 %
Thiamine	25 %
Riboflavin	25 %
Calcium	2 %
Iron	45 %
Vitamin D	10 %

How many bowls of cereal would you have to eat to meet the U.S. RDA for:

1. Vitamin A ?_____ 4 bowls _____

2. Protein ?_____ 20 bowls _____

3. Calcium ?_____ 50 bowls _____

What would be a better way to meet the U.S. RDA? Explain.

Eat a variety of foods from all the food groups

LABEL ABLE (DN-34)

DIRECTIONS: Refer to the Understanding Food Labels worksheet and answer the following questions:

1. How many *total* ounces of Grain Grungies Cereal are in a box? __**14.3 OUNCES**__

2. How many calories in a serving of Grain Grungies Cereal come from protein? __**12**__

3. How many calories come from carbohydrates? __**112**__

4. How many calories come from fat? __**18**__

5. Name the four minerals that Grain Grungies Cereal lists in the U.S. RDA:

   PHOSPHORUS
   MAGNESIUM
   ZINC
   COPPER

6. Is Grain Grungies Cereal considered a good fiber source? __**NO**__

7. Why or why not? __**It does not have 3 or more grams.**__

8. What ingredient in Grain Grungies Cereal is present in the largest amount? **CORN MEAL**

9. How do you know that? __**It is listed first in the ingredients.**__

©1993 by The Center for Applied Research in Education

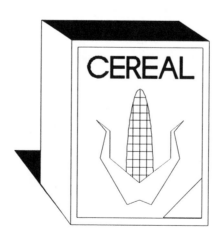

ADDITIVES OR PRESERVATIVES? (DN-38)

DIRECTIONS: If the boldface term in each sentence is correct, leave it as is. If it is **not** correct, cross it out and write the correct term in the space provided. All categories of additives are in the box below:

nutrients	**leavening agents**
preservatives	**pH control agents**
antioxidants	**emulsifiers**
humectants	**stabilizers**
anti-caking agents	**maturing and bleaching agents**

1. **Nutrients** are substances added to food to make it more nutritious, such as vitamins or minerals. _____

2. ~~**Texturizers**~~, such as citric acid and sorbic acid, help prevent food spoilage from microorganisms. **preservatives** _____

3. ~~**Emulsifiers**~~ delay and prevent rancidity or enzymatic browning. Examples are BHA and BHT. **antioxidants** _____

4. **Humectants** like sorbitol and glycerine cause foods to retain moisture. _____

5. ~~**Anti-caking agents**~~ affect cooking texture and volume. **leavening agents** _____

6. ~~**Leavening agents**~~ change and/or maintain acidity or alkalinity. **pH control agents** _____

7. Polysorbates and diglycerides are ~~**preservatives**~~ that help to keep liquids from separating. **emulsifiers** _____

8. **Stabilizers** improve texture, consistency, and body. _____

9. **Maturing and bleaching agents** improve baking qualities and accelerate the food aging process. _____

10. ~~**Humectants**~~ prevent caking and lumping. **anti-caking agents** _____

LET'S DO LUNCH! (DN-46)

DIRECTIONS: Look at the lunch below. Use the Food Cards (DN-40 to DN-45) to answer the questions in the box. Is this a nutritious lunch? Why or why not?

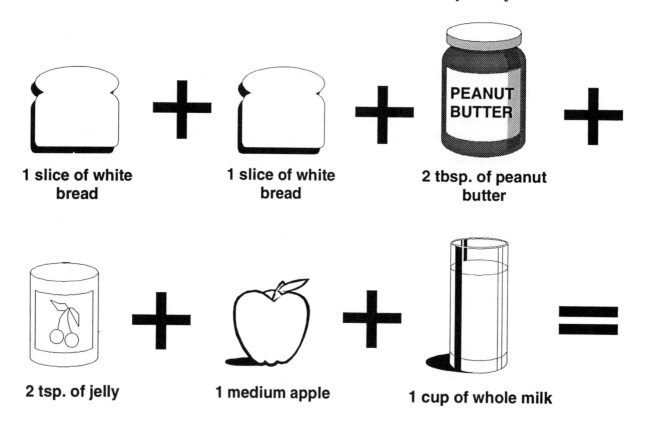

1 slice of white bread   +   1 slice of white bread   +   2 tbsp. of peanut butter   +

2 tsp. of jelly   +   1 medium apple   +   1 cup of whole milk   =

©1993 by The Center for Applied Research in Education

Total number of calories	582
Total grams of fat	26 grams
Total milligrams of cholesterol	33 milligrams
Total milligrams of sodium	536 milligrams
Total grams of protein	20 grams
Total grams of carbohydrates	71 grams

FOOD CARDS QUESTIONNAIRE (DN-47)

DIRECTIONS: Refer to the FOOD CARDS (DN-40 to DN-45) and answer the following
questions:

1. Which *group* of foods is highest in sodium? **Meat group**

2. Which food is highest in sodium? **Ham**

3. Which *group* of foods is lowest in carbohydrates? **Meat group**

4. Which *three groups* are very low in cholesterol? **Vegetable group**

   Grains group

   Fruit group

5. Which food is highest in cholesterol? **Hard-cooked egg**

6. Which food is lowest in calories? **Celery**

7. Which *two foods* are highest in calories? **Doughnut**

   Chocolate cake

8. Which vegetable is highest in carbohydrates? **Baked potato**

9. Which food from the meat group has the most fat? **Beef hot dog**

   How much? **17 grams**

10. Which food from the grains group is highest in sodium? **Cornflakes**

    Lowest? **Oatmeal**

THE AMERICAN DIET (DN-50)

DIRECTIONS: The graph below compares the average American diet with a diet recommended by many leading nutrition experts. Use the graph to answer the questions.

IN PERCENTAGES

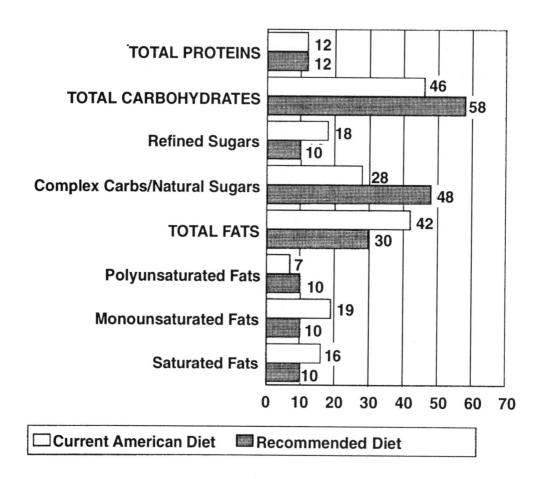

1. **What percentage of the American diet is made up of saturated fats?** _16%_
2. **What is recommended?** _10%_
3. **What percentage of the American diet is made up of all fats?** _42%_
4. **What is recommended?** _30%_
5. **What category remains the same for the current and recommended diets?** _Proteins_
6. **By how much does the recommended diet suggest that Americans cut their use of refined sugars?** _8%_
7. **By how much does the recommended diet suggest Americans increase complex carbohydrate consumption?** _20%_

CALORIES AND BMR (DN-64)

DIRECTIONS: Listed below is an explanation of basal metabolic rate (BMR) and how to estimate it for yourself. Figure your BMR and answer the questions.

Basal metabolic rate (BMR) is the rate at which you use energy when completely at rest. BMR varies according to age, sex, weight, and body size and shape. To get a rough estimate of your BMR in calories per day:

EXAMPLE (100-pound girl):

GIRLS:
1. Take your weight and add a zero: _____ 1000
2. Add your weight to that figure: + _____ +100
3. This is your approximate BMR: _____ 1,100 cal/day

EXAMPLE (150-pound boy)

BOYS:
1. Take your weight and add a zero: _____ 1500
2. Double your weight and add it: + _____ +300
3. This is your approximate BMR: _____ 1,800 cal/day

Calories are a measure of heat energy released when nutrients are burned or broken down. The more calories a food has, the more energy it contains. The number of calories a person needs in a day depends on many factors, such as amount of activity, air temperature, and BMR.

There are 3,500 calories in a pound of fat. To lose a pound, you would have to burn up 3,500 more calories than you consume. To gain a pound, you would have to eat 3,500 more calories than you burn.

---

1. How is it possible to have a high calorie/low nutrient diet?
   Junk food contains empty calories and few nutrients but is high in calories.

2. Does an active person need more or fewer calories per day? Explain.
   Yes. They need more calories per day to power the activities.

3. How might outside air temperature affect calorie burning?
   The colder the air temperature, the more calories you require to maintain a constant body temperature.

FITNESS OR FATNESS? QUIZ (DN-76)

DIRECTIONS: How much do you know about fitness? Take the quiz below by placing a *T* for true or an *F* for false in the blank.

F   1. To get the most benefits from exercising, it is necessary to exercise at least one hour every day.

(20 to 30 minutes three times per week is recommended by many experts.)

F   2. To increase the size of your leg muscles, you should lift weights every day to exercise the same group of muscles.

(Exercising the same muscle groups every day using weights is liable to cause injury.)

T   3. If you stop exercising, your present level of fitness will begin to drop after only one week of inactivity.

T   4. For static stretches to increase flexibility, they must be held for 15 to 20 seconds.

F   5. Women who lift weights will develop huge muscles and look masculine.

(Women lack large amounts of the male hormone testosterone, which is responsible for increased muscle size.)

F   6. It is best to eat sugar or sweets before competition to give yourself plenty of energy for a long period of time.

(Sugar actually can cause a brief increase but then hinder performance. Eat pasta or other complex carbohydrates instead.)

F   7. Take salt tablets when you exercise in hot weather.

(Extra salt does more harm than good and causes nausea and cramps.)

F   8. Don't drink water when working out; it can cause cramps.

(Always replace water when thirsty. Lack of water causes cramps).

T   9. It is better to eat a banana to replace potassium than to drink a sports drink before competition.

T   10. Target heart rate is 60% to 75% of your maximum heart rate and is the heart rate you should attain and stay at during an aerobic workout.

©1993 by The Center for Applied Research in Education

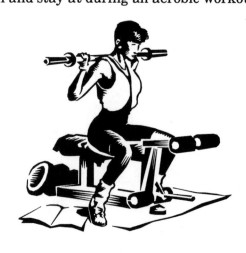

TRUE-FALSE DIETING QUIZ (DN-79)

DIRECTIONS: How much do you know about safe dieting? Place a *T* for true or an *F* for false in the blank to the left.

F   1. The body's need for food is far greater than its need for water.

T   2. Use the U.S. RDA to find the exact percentages of key nutrients you need.

T   3. Health experts recommend that you not lose more than 1½ pounds to 2 pounds per week when on a diet.

T   4. People who are extremely underweight can have as many problems as people who are overweight.

F   5. If you eat more calories than you burn, you will lose weight.

F   6. There are 1000 calories in one pound of fat.

T   7. Even a small amount of exercise can help speed up your metabolic rate.

F   8. When you diet, the first weight to be lost will be fat.

F   9. The pinch test and skin caliper test are used to measure the amount of muscle under the skin.

T   10. Diuretics are medications that cause the body to lose water weight.

EATING DISORDERS: Anorexia Nervosa (DN-81)

DIRECTIONS: Research the eating disorder Anorexia Nervosa and answer the questions.

1. What is ANOREXIA NERVOSA?

Anorexia is a behavior involving the irrational fear of becoming overweight and results in severe weight loss from starvation.

2. What are some of the possible causes?

Obsession with thinness, psychological pressures, and problems; may be due to low self-concept, inability to cope, outside pressures, high expectations, the need to achieve, the need for attention, or the unconscious desire to remain a child.

3. What are the signs and symptoms?

Low calorie intake (500 to 800 calories per day), great interest in food, obsessive intense exercising, fear of obesity even when underweight, inaccurate body image, attitude of extreme perfectionism, extreme weight loss, denial of an eating problem, absence of menstrual periods in females, hormone changes resulting in downy hair on the back and chest, constipation, emotional problems.

4. What are the health risks?

Body is deprived of essential nutrients, severe malnutrition, hair loss, organ damage, death from heart problems or suicide.

5. Where, in your community, can you get help for eating disorders?

Answers will vary.

EATING DISORDERS: Bulimia (DN-82)

DIRECTIONS: Research the eating disorder BULIMIA and answer the questions.

1. What is BULIMIA?

Bulimia is an episodic pattern of binge eating that involves rapid consumption of a large quantity of food in a short time followed by self-induced vomiting or diarrhea.

2. What are some of the possible causes?

The desire to become thin, the desire to be more attractive, the desire for physical perfection, the fear of being out of control.

3. What are the signs and symptoms?

Excessive eating followed by self-induced vomiting, use of laxatives, enemas, and diuretics to lose weight, impulsive and often socially unacceptable behavior, tooth decay, absence of menstrual periods, dehydration, depression and mood swings, constant pursuit of thinness.

4. What are the health risks?

Protein-calorie malnutrition, dehydration, hypokalemia (low potassium in the blood), dental enamel erosion, vitamin and mineral deficiency; possible organ damage, internal bleeding from vomiting, possibility of cardiovascular and kidney failure.

5. Where, in your community, can you get help for eating disorders?

Answers will vary.

NUTRITION CROSSWORD PUZZLE (DN-85)

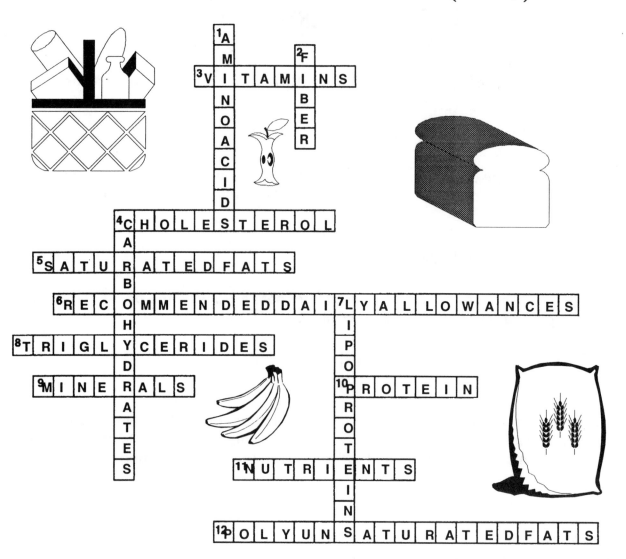

DOWN

1. Building blocks of protein
2. The nondigestible part of certain foods that aids in moving food through the digestive tract
4. Chemical compounds that are converted to glycogen when broken down during digestion
7. Special molecules that carry cholesterol through the bloodstream

ACROSS

3. Organic compounds that work with enzymes to promote chemical changes
4. Fatty substance found in all animal tissue
5. Fatty acid with as many hydrogen atoms as it can hold
6. A general guide to the amount of nutrients needed daily
8. Three fatty acids attached to one glycerol molecule
9. Inorganic substances formed in the earth with distinct chemical and physical properties
10. The second most abundant substance in the human body and a vital part of every cell
11. Chemical substances obtained from food during digestion
12. Fatty acid that has room for four or more hydrogen atoms

NUTRITION MATCH-UP (DN-86)

DIRECTIONS: Match the correct term with its definition by placing the correct letter in the blank to the left. Not all terms will be used.

k 1. Losing and gaining weight repeatedly

r 2. A unit of energy

n 3. Serious illness from overeating and self-induced vomiting

b 4. Abnormal loss of body fluids

h 5. Eating plan that requires cutting down on salt

i 6. Eating plan limiting foods high in animal and other saturated fats

g 7. Last date a product should be used

a 8. Bacteria found in improperly canned foods that can cause illness and death

c 9. Foods relatively low in fat

p 10. Food that uses the entire kernel and contains most of the original nutrients

a. botulism
b. dehydration
c. chicken, turkey (skinless)
d. beef, pork
e. nutrition label
f. unit pricing
g. expiration date
h. low-sodium diet
i. low-cholesterol diet
j. setpoint
k. yo-yo dieting
l. crash dieting
m. anorexia
n. bulimia
o. perfringen poisoning
p. whole wheat bread
q. white bread
r. calorie

CROSSED UP! (DN-87)

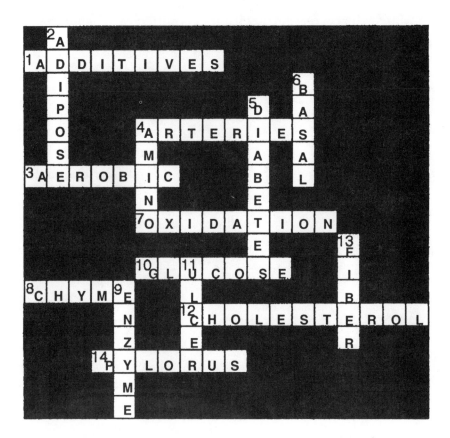

ACROSS

1. Substances added to food
3. Exercise that increases oxygen intake to stimulate the heart and lungs
4. Blood vessels that carry blood from the heart to the body
7. Process by which cells use oxygen to turn food into energy
8. Mixture of gastric juices and food in the stomach
10. Blood sugar
12. Substance found in blood, tissues, and digestive juices, too much of which can cause heart disease
14. A muscle that separates the stomach from the small intestine

DOWN

2. Body cells that store fat
4. Protein building blocks: _____ acids
5. Illness where the pancreas does not make enough insulin
6. The rate at which the body uses energy for it's basic processes: _____ metabolic rate (BMR)
9. Substance that speeds up a chemical process
11. Stomach sore
13. Carbohydrate found in plant foods that helps the digestive system work more smoothly